Spaciousness
The Radical Dzogchen of the Vajra-Heart
Longchenpa's *Treasury of the Dharmadhatu*

Other Titles by Keith Dowman

For digital information please visit: www.keithdowman.net

Spaciousness

The Radical Dzogchen of the Vajra-Heart

Longchenpa's *Treasury of the Dharmadhatu*

Translation from the Tibetan and Commentary
Keith Dowman

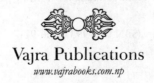

Vajra Publications
www.vajrabooks.com.np

Published by

Vajra Publications

Jyatha, Thamel, Kathmandu, Nepal
Tel.: 977-1-4220562, Fax: 977-1-4246536
e-mail: bidur_la@mos.com.np
www.vajrabooks.com.np

Distributed by

Vajra Books

Kathmandu, Nepal

ISBN 978-9937-506-97-7

Printed in Nepal

Dedicated to
all sentient beings that they may realize
the great perfection in all its clarity,
freedom and compassion.

Contents

Contents

Preface

This translation may appear to some readers as a finished work of English composition reflecting Longchenpa's Tibetan original. This is far from the truth. Longchenpa's *Treasury of the Dharmadhatu* is a masterpiece of poetic mystical revelation and requires a mind of similar luminosity to render it into English. Longchenpa's major works comprise only a fraction of the mystical masterpieces of Tibetan Buddhism that require translation with a pitch of resonance and height of evocation similar to the King James' version of the bible. We need western Longchenpas to rewrite this perennial mystical experience in an authentic language ringing true from the first word to the last. We have expunged a lot of the tired English argot that was contrived originally to translate the Mahayana sutras and shastras, but we still have a long way to go before Dzogchen texts shine in the great tradition of English poetry and of T.S. Eliot or Jack Kerouac – and it is the poetry that matters as much as, or even more than, the philosophical content. The academics are necessary and useful, but our best hope for Dzogchen texts lies with the yogin-poets, even if that implies expanding the scope of transmission to include a far wider audience.

Does this approach vitiate the lineage in any way? Does it permit unscrupulous charlatan or psychopathic teachers to preempt the closed circle of Dzogchen lineage-holders in a susceptible, credulous, new age market? What of the new-age Dzogchen imitators who have obtained their knowledge from books and study? Should they be welcomed as homegrown, self-realized, nondualist Dzogchen adepts? "Lineage" in Dzogchen is synonymous with "the ground of being", but is it the *sine qua non* for other nondual teachers? And then the issue of samaya: we must accept that subsequent to initiatory experience, until a student has assimilated and familiarized him or herself with the view, secrecy

– or at least discretion – can be extremely valuable as a hedge against energy leakage and conventional, deleterious prioritization. Yet, since the heart-teaching is always self-secret, dissemination of the Dzogchen view and celebration of the great significance of nonmeditation need not be circumscribed by the teacher's personal vow of secrecy. Due to poor presentation some recipients of the view may find their egos inflated by it; but for most recipients the view is ego-destructive and undermines and resolves the manipulative, dualizing intellect.

This is another, alternative, translation of the seminal Dzogchen text *Chos dbyings mdzod*, which is the Tibetan master Longchenpa's masterpiece. The first publication of this work, in 2001, under the title *The Precious Treasury of Basic Space,* may yet prove to be a turning point in the history of Dzogchen in the West. A group of western Dzogchen practitioners, who had not absorbed Dzogchen in its oriental home, translated and published the supreme classical work of Dzogchen under the auspices of a rigzin-lama and with the assistance of khenpo-scholars, but essentially inspired by their own existential understanding. Dzogchen was thus reclaimed by the people who need it from the caretakers who can no longer use it in the cultural context in which it evolved. Surely we should hope that Dzogchen retains a deep sacred place within Tibetan consciousness, but our principal aspiration is for Dzogchen to take root in the West and heal the deep rifts that Judeo-Christian dualism has created in the meta-structural consciousness of the People of the Book. In order for this to occur, the supra-cultural meaning of Dzogchen should be lifted by its existential bootstraps out of its monastic isolation and primping cultishness into the clear light of day, where it can be embraced by the existential and literary mainstream that is open to a nondual view of the world. This translation attempts to move literary Dzogchen exposition in that direction.

Dzogchen must leap out of the academies into the lives of the people on the ground who aspire to live it, or, rather, who are struggling to live it as through a glass darkly without the benefit of the heart-teaching. Governed now by an elitist group of linguists and sectarian, commercial publishers on one side and covens of secretive esoteric practitioners on the other, Dzogchen risks becoming lost in an impenetrable sectarian labyrinth. The religious history of Tibet had its own necessary religio-political logic that banished Dzogchen to a secret, underground status; the needs of the West surely require quite a different upshot.

Longchenpa's work, like this one, allows the possibility that scientists, the high priests of a post-Christian society, particularly the physicists, can recognize the apex of Buddhist thinking as a corollary of their own. Dzogchen texts and western commentaries should be accessible to psychologists – particularly cognitive psychiatrists and Gestalt psychologists – to physicists, particularly particle and quantum physicists, and philosophers. From East Asia, Zen, Ch'an and Taoism have created a profound wave of spacious, inseminating attitudes and vibration flooding through the thinking of many western disciplines – Dzogchen is set to crown that tendency. A similar statement could be made about the influence of Advaita Vedanta and Kashmiri Shaivism upon the West; but Dzogchen will eclipse their influence because of the breadth of its view, the rationality and scope of its mysticism, the lucidity and clarity of its texts and the deep roots and vitality of its tradition.

Not only should scholars be released and absolved from their stranglehold on Dzogchen exposition, but the conservatism of Tibetan holders of the tradition should also be given a rest. As conservators of the Vajrayana tradition in general, and Dzogchen in particular, the Tibetan rigzins and tulkus could not be surpassed. Even the holocaust of the Chinese Cultural Revolution could not destroy what they had preserved in scripture and in oral transmission for as much as twelve hundred years. Now, in the exile environment, limited nationalistic thinking may defeat the purpose of their dharma when non-Tibetan people hungry for the vital meaning of nondualism need the transmission so urgently. This assumes that the Dzogchen mindset goes a long way to resolving the world's ecological, political and economic problems. It would be tragic indeed if Dzogchen were to remain the exclusive prerogative of those with birthright and thereby allow it to perish within the inevitable death throes of autochthonous Tibetan religious culture. What western consumers of Dzogchen require from the Tibetan lamas are the qualities that Dzogchen espouses – detachment, openness, spontaneity, kindness and an inclusive supportive fellowship. With condescension, self-serving or tightfisted protectiveness, or an acquisitive business attitude, the bud on the bough is likely to wither before spring is out. Like economic protectionism, spiritual isolationism is counter-productive, like shooting oneself in the foot. As a codicil to that, I reflect that my own root gurus, although sustaining a genuine front of traditionalism, in my perception were infinitely flexible, bountifully generous and graciously supportive – but that was at an earlier, more humbling, more auspicious time.

In conclusion, we congratulate Richard Barron for his groundbreaking translations of Longchenpa's *Seven Treasuries* and honor Chagdud Tulku among Tibetans for his rare faith in his western disciples' understanding and realization. Just as a crystal once grown in an experimental laboratory can thereafter more easily be grown in another far distant laboratory, so once a text has been opened by one translator it is made immensely more accessible to others. If Dzogchen is Tibet's greatest gift to humanity those who can should work together to share it without stint.

Keith Dowman
The Great Stupa
Boudha, Kathmandu
Losar, Water Snake: 2013

Introduction

This famous seminal text of radical Dzogchen provides a profound yet simple poetic statement of how it is to immerse oneself in the matrix of the now, to allow pure presence and recognize buddha. It is a personal statement of a yogin-adept who, evidently, has passed through the throes of transfiguration. Certainly the magic of his poetry impresses us that way and surely this *Treasury of the Dharmadhatu,* the *Choyingdzo,* is a personal revelation of the consummation of Dzogchen. In it we are assured that over and above all the yogas and dhyanas of Hindustan, all the ritual and magic of Tibet and all the commercialized quasi-religious new-age therapies of the West there exists a simple, timeless manner of being, of easy access, requiring no onerous technique or renunciate lifestyle, that can give us a constant modicum of satisfaction in this vale of tears between birth and dying.

This magnum opus of Longchen Rabjampa is a textbook of what has become known as radical Dzogchen, so called in distinction to latter-day elaborated Dzogchen. It is a root text of those who have come up through the ranks of Buddhist practice, and that includes most Tibetans who are familiar with it and most westerners who have prior meditation experience on the graduated path. Even more so it is a textbook for those who have encountered Buddhism at this its apex point through the instruction of those few lamas who promote Dzogchen distinct from its Buddhist context or who have had personal, initiatory experience outside any institutional frame. Its clarity in pointing out the natural great perfection is unsurpassed. Its absence of pedantry and didacticism and its fullness of poetic diction make it a paean of personal revelation, a naked revelation of a buddha-yogin-cum-poet.

The Tibetan Vajrayana Buddhist arena historically is riven in a multitude of ways. Between the four schools, for instance, and between the old and new propagations, between monastic and lay practitioners, between the shamanic and the reformist, between central and eastern provinces, and not least in significance is the gap between monastic academics and lay yogins. To appreciate these two extremes of life-style and attitude compare Je Tsongkhapa, the great Gelukpa literary exponent of the monastic reformist tradition, with Drukpa Kunley, the wandering Buddhist sadhu (ngakpa), minstrel, magician, philanderer – and Dzogchen adept and poet. No love is lost between these two modes of spiritual exemplar, a tendency that has carried over to the West, where both Tibetan and, particularly, some western academics pour militant scorn upon their experientially inspired, more demonstrative and less intellectual brothers. The monks who were the butt of his teaching-jokes basted Drukpa Kunley. Of course, academics talk while yogins walk the dharma, and academics extol and cultivate the very faculty that Dzogchen yogins seek to deflate and mitigate. Arrogance is the natural corollary of intellectual accomplishment, while humility arises automatically in the adept's mind through his unfurnished lifestyle. But as Dudjom Rinpoche famously advised, the Dzogchen adept must be alert to the danger of attachment to alcohol and fornication.

That academics as well as adepts have enormously enriched Tibetan culture is indisputable. What needs to be stressed is that the apex of Vajrayana exposition is revealed where yoga as existential accomplishment and literary exposition as poetry coincide. This middle-way place, halfway between monastery and chung-house-cum-brothel, is the hermitage, not so much a place of rigorous ascetic discipline as a place of spiritual freedom. Here we can find the finest analytic and expressive minds and the very broad and profound all-inclusive view incorporated in the single embodiment that is buddha. Saraha exalted the tradition in India; Milarepa was buddha, a Tibetan of the Himalayan littoral; another – and in the Dzogchen tradition the finest – was Longchenpa. *The Treasury of the Dharmadhatu* is the most explicit and keenest of the expositions of his own experience of Dzogchen atiyoga. He himself stresses the personal nature of what he describes. The real Dzogchen experience is beyond description and expression so what he writes is of course a personal elaboration.

This all-inclusive view that is the reality of radical Dzogchen is not dependent upon any religious culture, although the priests of the Buddhist and Bon religions of Tibet have been the custodians and occasional exemplars of it. For that we owe them an enormous debt of gratitude, which is now being repaid by patrons and disciples in the dharma-centers throughout the world, and an even greater debt for investing us in the West in their vital tradition, repaid by our recognition of the nature of mind. But radical Dzogchen is, after all, as the tradition affirms, what we have always known. We know the inimical truth of being along with all human beings who listen to their deep heart's core and at the same time open their eyes to what is there in front of their faces. We know it in the same way that we know the pulsing of the blood in our veins and the touch of the inbreath and the outbreath on our nostrils. The truth of Dzogchen is the legacy of being human. But Judeo-Christian theism and Manichean dualism have persistently obstructed such direct knowledge, nondualism proscribed as heretical, and Christian culture has never been able to articulate it sufficiently to create an integral lineal tradition, either covert or secular. Nevertheless, the nondual reality of Dzogchen shines through European literature and poetry by other means. It is evident in popular culture – or is it most particularly evident in pop culture? – and the truth dawns that it is the heartbeat of all culture. By virtue of the counter-cultural revolution of the sixties, moreover, insofar as the communal mind was opened and made receptive to the profound blast of radical Dzogchen, today we have access to texts such as those of Longchenpa, each containing an identical vision, like pixels in a hologram, that simultaneously mirror and irradiate disparate visions in the minds of innumerable people around the world.

The yoga of the vajra-heart, Maha-Ati, the apex path, is not part of the ninefold schema of progressive Nyingma Buddhism and yet it infuses all nine aspects. Longchenpa introduces it as an ultimately transcendent view that lies outside the narrative of the nine paths and outside the conventional frame that includes atiyoga. In so doing he provides a rationale for the perception of Dzogchen independent of its Buddhist context, a separable and discrete discipline. Such a perspective is key to the radical Dzogchen view; the recognition of the nature of mind is predicated upon the introduction from a master, whether he is a Buddhist or Bon rigzin-lama, and regardless of his religious faith or whether indeed he is of a religious or secular disposition. On the other hand, in some cantos within this poem, Longchenpa appears to identify the apex view with atiyoga, the ninth path. The distinction here is to be made between instantaneous Dzogchen perceived as simultaneous starting point and destination, wherein no gradation within a space-time frame can be admitted, and Dzogchen as a short – momentary – path, a doorway into the nature of mind in space-time.

At its essence atiyoga may be conceived as either trekcho or togal, the two slightly differing facets of Dzogchen. The question whether the apex view is identical to the trekcho and togal views is one of those false questions posed by the intellect as a last defense against ego-loss. If this question prepossesses us, we need to fall back into the spaciousness of the thought and allow the nonduality of nonaction to reassert itself. If the intellect, rejecting that response as a placebo, insists on a rational answer to the question "Why?" when the Dzogchen view insists that there is nothing to do, do we need to engage with the techniques of trekcho and togal? Again the answer is "nonaction". But what, then, of the outer and the inner preliminary practices and the trekcho and togal nonmeditations? What of the formulations of the view under which *The Treasury of the Dharmadhatu* could be subsumed? Yes, the vajra-heart is the immediate recourse of those who, like the great garuda bird, spread their wings upon hatching, take off into the azure sky and never look back. Atiyoga, conversely, is the treasury of concepts and modalities that are the wide-open doorways to serendipitous integration. In order to fall into the self-sprung understanding that the distinction between relative and absolute is purely intellectual and delusive, there must be a concept, a doorway, that is understood as nondual. That concept, and others denominated by its synonyms, is understood as a doorway into nonduality. The experience of walking through the door is like opening a door to the outside and allowing the air outside to merge with the air inside. While having the eyes open and looking, it is the experience of suddenly seeing. While dreaming, it is the sudden recognition that we are dreaming. So long as these exercises and concepts are considered functions of nonaction and thus doorways into the nondual, we remain in the realm of radical Dzogchen. The moment that any technique is conceived as a method providing a cause or condition for the realization of the natural state of mind, we enter the progressive, gradualist – cultural – path that is usually taught by the lineal protagonists of latter-day Dzogchen to those they believe cannot comprehend the rigorous precepts of radical Dzogchen. Longchenpa himself is indeed sitting in the cockpit of the vajra-heart, sitting astride the great garuda, and presenting the apex view as the only ultimately valid perspective, but he has practiced all the nine approaches to which the Nyingma tradition subscribes. He calls them "lesser" or "lower" because the practitioners of those paths are caught up in the form – view, meditation technique and lifestyle – of those disciplines and thus nurse themselves into a purgatory of limitations where they can only await the ultimate, synchronicitous transmission. The nine Buddhist paths are succinct metaphors designed for various embodied mindsets to gradually (or in the case of the ninth path immediately) extricate themselves from the delusion of being separate entities. Thus, they are only relatively valid, and valid most particularly where Buddhist cultural mores and Buddhist tradition mold the culture, especially in the tantric context where lifestyle, culture and meditation are inextricably entangled and least valid where assumptions about the nature of reality are not derived from Hindu mysticism. In the West, we may winnow the chaff of oriental Buddhist culture until we have an essence of Theravada monastic praxis or bodhisattva householder morality, for instance, but Buddhist monasteries and Buddhist monks stick out like sore thumbs in our post-Christian culture. For these reasons, if the reader lives enmeshed in a football-and-beer culture he need not trouble himself about the occasional comment in Longchenpa's text alluding to the nine lower approaches. Unless there is timorousness in the face of the essential spaciousness or emptiness of the cultural charade, we do not need kind and sympathetic, gradualist, Buddhist culture in order to enter the Dzogchen mandala. And for these reasons, however, the core vitality of Buddhism – the Dzogchen – remains sequestered, the prerogative of scholars playing semantic games and academic one-upmanship.

In order to reach the plane where there is no ladder of spirituality to climb and no pyramid of meditational accomplishment to hold us in awe, we need to be free of the notion that we can fall to a lower level of existential cognizance or rise to any higher state. Only then can we relax into the all-embracing matrix of the now. Culturally based practices produce progressive cultural accomplishment. The nature of mind abhors structures of any kind, says Longchenpa, but particularly, he might add, those that are constructed through ambition, competition and contention reinforcing the sense of self. Thus it is tempting to believe that when Longchenpa was alive, in the fourteenth century, the phases of recognition of mind's nature to which the terms "trekcho" and "togal" refer were still aspects of the same unitary noncausal Dzogchen atiyoga praxis. It appears that by the eighteenth century the gradualists had come to dominate the Nyingma School overtly, no doubt strongly influenced by the Gelukpa establishment in Lhasa. Thereafter, trekcho and togal were the highest two rungs on a Dzogchen ladder. Both the latter-day dominant lineages carrying Dzogchen transmission – the Longchen Nyingtik and Kunzang Gongpa Zangtal traditions – demonstrate this. Although the vajra-heart was still beating fast, the cultural, relativist aspect was dominant. Here in *The Treasury of the Dharmadhatu*, a textbook of radical Dzogchen, the single use of each term – trekcho and togal – clearly defines their original meanings as aspects of an identical experience. Trekcho is the phase or aspect of the resolution of duality where the luminous mind shines through as alpha-purity, as primordial awareness. Togal is the phase or aspect of the same resolution where that same luminous mind is perceived in a unitary experience of spontaneously arising phenomena. The proposition that the one necessarily precedes the other merely shows the intellectual propensity that enforces causal interconnection. Or perhaps the canard of causal succession arose when trekcho and togal became associated with different practices in the process of developing gradualism, where preliminary exercises were connected to trekcho. Thus instead of relating like two sides of the same coin, trekcho and togal flowed one after the other in the gradualist practitioner's process as basic practice and fruition, as cause and effect.

It is sometimes asserted that specifically trekcho practices develop the empty aspect of reality experientially, while togal practices develop the form, and in the exposition of the progressive path this distinction seems to be generally accepted. Yet the intellect that separated trekcho and togal is the same faculty that is now separating emptiness and appearances. Is it beneficial to assume that these two can be separated in any way – existentially – in the now? Is it useful to conceive of successive development of the poles of this dualism? To develop one is of course to develop the other, and anyway what is this notion of development? Is Dzogchen a progressive, graduated path after all?

Might there be benefit in polishing or upgrading the ego? In the vajra-heart we have left all concepts of a spiritual path and spiritual praxis behind. Indeed radical Dzogchen can be distinguished by its separation from all goal-orientated practices and that includes, particularly, the eight lower of the nine approaches of the Nyingma system. Strictly, the radical Dzogchen path is a formless path and therefore may be called a pathless path. As direct experience of a unified field it is the prerogative of an elite – but not an intellectual elite. On the contrary, insofar as our culture tends to reward those with acutely rational intellects, even more so than in the past, a tendency towards enshrining intellectual dialectics enthralls us, and that is impossible in radical Dzogchen, because the trekcho practices have undermined causality. If intellectual arrogance raises its ugly head, it is the demonic head of ego assuming that there is a goal, near or far, that needs to be accomplished and that there is a technique, the prerogative of superior intellect, that can accomplish it.

What is crucial in this vajra-heart scenario? What is the key to pure presence? The crux is the place where dualities are resolved, where mind is never distracted or drawn away; it has no motivation and remains in its natural disposition, transcending all goal-orientation. At that place lies the crucial recognition of intrinsic spaciousness itself; resting therein, whatever arises naturally subsides, vanishing, released just as it is, without effort. Afflictive emotion, karma and habitual propensities, and even methods of improvement on the path of liberation, arise as illusory magical display from creativity; everything arises in the now as a display of creativity and it is only recognized just as it is without any modification. No matter what situation arises, we do not engage in it in order to improve it or to try to suppress it, for the key to pure presence is freely resting in our natural disposition. Thus nonaction is the key and the crux. In the Dzogchen view nonaction is recognized as noncausality, nonduality, unitary sameness, indivisibility and immediacy. If we gain familiarity with the luminous essence – the luminous spontaneity of things – through the key precept of nonstriving and effortlessness, buddha in the now is buddha reawakened. It is the actuality of the peerless vajra-heart – the essence of the ninefold path that is the luminous supermatrix. Phantasmagoria self-releasing, reality is consummate Dzogchen, and invariable spontaneity is the crux of this excellent counsel of Longchenpa.

Dzogchen surely has a life independent of Buddhism, but the truth of Sakyamuni's fundamental insights often shines through the precepts of Dzogchen's radical existentialism. Each stanza of *The Treasury of the Dharmadhatu* may be considered a precept, or a nest of precepts, and in the satisfaction of unpacking them Buddhist sutric insights are renewed. Giving attention for the duration of an experience of pure presence (rigpa), for example, lost in the awareness of the constant flux inherent in the natural reality of spontaneity, the notion of "impermanence" becomes experiential. What appears to have some permanence, however, persists for a period not just shorter in duration than a fraction of a nanosecond, but for no extension in time whatsoever. Further, impermanence is connoted in the adjective "self-sprung" when it qualifies "pristine awareness". The indulgent associations of "continuum" are only allowed in "the continuum of discursive opinion", for example, and also regarding the process of constant change when objects deflate instantaneously, dissolving in nonmeditation. The ephemeral nature of reality is best experienced simply by dwelling in the now; realization of the transitory nature of the illusion that fills experience is thus burnt indelibly into consciousness. Then "signlessness", one of the three doors to liberation, central to sutric Buddhism, is an attribute of Dzogchen experience emphasized and reiterated in trekcho – although it is emphasized less in togal where discovery of evidence of pure presence in the visual field is paramount. Then, "selflessness" likewise is implicit in the Dzogchen view, although it is rarely overtly stated as such unless the repetition of "apparent but nonexistent", usually referring to the objective illusion of something insubstantial, is construed as an affirmation of the nonexistence of any subjective self. We gain an impression throughout *The Treasury of the Dharmadhatu* that Longchenpa's witness has long retired.

Whereas the perspective on reality presented by the various Buddhist paths and meditations (excluding Dzogchen) stimulates the motivation to strive on the path of moral and cognitive purification, it is imperative to understand that this poem is in no way a prescription upon which to act. It describes "what is" on a very deep existential level and thus provokes recognition of that "reality". To believe what is being evoked is a higher, better, state of being than what we have now and, therefore, something that we should espouse and commit ourselves to and work towards, is to make self-abuse the purpose and basis of the Dzogchen view. Self-improvement and transformation are the trademarks of Buddhist tantra (Vajrayana); the Dzogchen view to the contrary implies reflexive recognition of the spaciousness of the timeless moment. The satisfaction that we may receive from visualizing the actuality of spaciousness and the nondual vision, to allow the intellect to turn it into a kind of existential delicacy that we may feast on occasionally if we do the correct ritual and liturgical oblation, is a self-defeating obstruction. On the treadmill of goal-orientation, inevitably our gold is transmuted into lead, or, rather, inexorably the gold dust in the palm of the hand trickles through the fingers and vanishes on the breeze. The guru-vision cannot become a goal or technique; if it becomes obsessive it reinforces the neurosis that is creating the pain and anxiety. Either we recognize the now outside of time or no recognition is possible. Either we recognize the nature of mind or we are left with just an intellectual reflection, a representation or repackaging of direct perception.

For many and various reasons it is crucial to understand that this poem is not a philosophical treatise. If philosophy is the theoretical study of knowledge and existence, Dzogchen is not a philosophy since Dzogchen is preeminently experiential. If philosophy is a love of wisdom for its own sake, again that is not Dzogchen, but more of an indulgence in the realm of pure form where we can take uninhibited pleasure in appreciation of abstract relations as in mathematics or music. In that space we would take pleasure in the complex and radical patterns of thought that create an existential net across the universe. Dzogchen is not another Buddhist blueprint for the understanding of the relative mind, part of a metapsychology that can optimize human potential or cure humanity of its ills. Nor does it provide a route to power and manipulation of other beings, nor power and technology to control the external world. Those who study Dzogchen as an academic discipline are like fearful nestlings looking over the edge of the nest aware that their wings still lack strength. Or perhaps they resemble fish pulled in on a line and having lost the ocean that is their natural medium are left to thrash about in the bottom of the boat. To treat Dzogchen like an integrated philosophy or a subject of study and analysis is to demonstrate ignorance that the Dzogchen view is a nondual view, the unity of the subject/object dichotomy; that there can be no dogma, doctrine or set practice in radical Dzogchen; that an analytical, intellectual approach adds sand to the tank that was to provide the fuel for the journey; that it hardens the arteries whose pliability and elasticity was our best hope for extra vitality. On the contrary Dzogchen is a yoga – the ultimate yoga – that provides, simply, the keys to authentic being.

Since Dzogchen is neither a philosophy nor a subject for academic analysis or comparison, we may eschew academic language and get rid of the diction that makes it appear sophistic. To translate what in Tibetan is understood as reality by the phrase "the true nature of phenomena", for example, is like taking a musty piece of archaic painted pottery out of a museum and using it to serve wine at a contemporary cocktail party. We do not need to brush off dignified and pretentious phrases from the history of Buddhist philosophy in order to describe the reality of being here and now. The alternative of course is to create a new language, a language of existential poetry. The structure and vocabulary of the language should itself reflect the nuance of its message – like haiku or koan or the siddhas' dohas. This is not so much a paean in praise of the style of this present translation but rather a statement of intent and a plea for Dzogchen translators of a new generation to get out of the rut of classical Buddhist diction.

Furthermore, Dzogchen is not a religion. The rites that are performed by Dzogchen communities are the legacy of the Buddhist or Bon religions by which Dzogchen has been transmitted. Recitation of mantra and visualization of deities, oblation, praise and prayer are all remnants of Buddhist tantra. Any ritual worship and dogma that are practiced by Dzogchen adepts have an extraneous source. Dzogchen cannot become a subject of comparative religion because it is not a religion any more than digging a garden is a religion, or maintaining a motorbike is a religion. Dzogchen is as natural as the beating of the heart or breathing through the nose. It is like walking down the razor's edge on a pathless path.

Dzogchen is an existential yoga and it can only be appreciated, criticized, and understood by living it, much as chocolate can only be known by tasting it. To those readers who are already nestled in the Dzogchen reality, Longchenpa's thirteen cantos may appear like a fishing net cast into an empty boat from the ocean, rather than a net cast into the sea from a boat replete with its catch. The fish are where they should be already – swimming with us in our sea; the boat, the fishermen and the net are redundant. To reiterate the simplistic traditional simile, why search in the jungle for the elephant when the animal is tied up in its stable? To those reading this in expectation of finding an answer to a the plight of separateness and alienation, to the eternal problem of suffering embodied in samsara, and thus exercising the rational analytic mind to unravel the conundrum of Dzogchen expression, consider the rainbow present in the dissolution of our elemental, corporeal body where resolution is attained. For those who trawl Longchenpa's cantos for a breath of fresh air, for a straw to hang on to as a life raft, the book should be thrown away, and in simply sitting the Dzogchen contemplation should be allowed to occur. Longchenpa does offer a solution to people strangled by their intellect in an era where society has not a jot of compassion for those of its members who have lost their intuitive sense of the unity of all things. His answer is to be found in the spaciousness of the nature of being that is the underlying, intrinsic, reality of the intellect, rather than in the cooperative meaning of his well-ordered words.

The taste of this existential yoga is expressed in verse, in thirteen cantos. A canto is a song and these thirteen songs are like thirteen planets revolving around a sun of the purest light, while the cantos' stanzas are like facets of each planet. Each of the cantos reflects an aspect of the central reality; the cantos' titles are all synonyms of the reality that is the ineffable sun. Likewise, each of the stanzas of the cantos is like a facet of a jewel, each reflecting the nature of mind, each in a different way. Expectation of a train of stanzas each linked one to the other by a linear thread of causal meaning developing from an hypothesis to a resolution will be disappointed, and construing a serial connection from stanza to stanza will be counterproductive. Each stanza is complete in itself, like each moment of pure presence in the now. While each stanza has a distinct cast providing a slightly different angle on the nature of mind, all the stanzas are the same. They are all the same in that what is evoked is always precisely the same thing. Likewise, the words themselves, although indicating superficially discrete meaning and the grammatical structure providing separate ontological status, they are all identical in the nature of mind.

The move away from expectation of graduated goal-oriented development to multi-faceted appreciation of the text parallels diminution of hope and fear of attaining goals in the future and its replacement by the realization of the perfection of the moment in all its multifarious variety.

Thirteen is a perfect number in the numerology of pre-buddhist Tibetan religion. Each of the thirteen cantos of this book presents a metaphysical formula that describes in its entirety a perspective upon reality. When every reference point in any given perspective is existentially deconstructed (pixelated), then differentiated, dualistic and conflicted constructs along with conjunct karmic propensities resolve themselves like horizontal lines of identically-colored squares disappearing in a game of Tetris, or vertical lines of cards of similar suit vanishing in a digital game of patience, and a unitary view results. The thirteen cantos therefore are like magic spells that evoke a single nondual view, the unitary Dzogchen view.

For those who need analytic supports to understand the cantos, if we construe the thirteen chapters according to a conventional structure and try to perceive serial development in the text, and in blocks of similar cantos, we can begin with the analysis of the scholar Nyoshul Lungtok. According to him, the first nine cantos are exposition of view, the tenth canto is on meditation, the eleventh on conduct, the twelfth on immediate results and the thirteenth on final results. Evidently, Nyoshul Lungtok was an academic belonging to the gradualist persuasion. Again, if we relate the thirteen cantos to the four samayas and trekcho and togal, the first five cantos relate to the first two samayas and trekcho, while the remaining seven cantos treat the second and third samayas and togal. Specifically the chapter entitled Spaciousness relates to absence and to openness; the chapter entitled Spontaneity relates to the third samaya; and Inclusivity and Nonduality relate to the fourth. Dzogchen disdains concepts; so are these differentiations useful? At least, most gradualists are unanimous in failing to find in *The Treasury of the Dharmadhatu* evidence that Longchenpa was more indebted to any one of the three series of Dzogchen (mind, matrix and secret precept series) rather than any other.

The lengthy commentary composed perhaps by Longchenpa's White Skull Mountain atelier provides further rational light upon *The Treasury of the Dharmadhatu*. It is not, however, the type of commentary that progresses word by word, phrase by phrase, or even stanza by stanza, elaborating the meaning. Rather, it provides a deep elaboration of meaning while utilizing the stanzas as pegs upon which to hang innumerable Dzogchen precepts indicating view and meditation. This information and instruction provide a first line of retreat from the immediate to the progressive perspective. In so doing, it reduces the majesty of Longchenpa's poetry to prosaic rational comment and the ultimacy of his meaning sometimes to avuncular advice, reducing the apex view and meditation of noncausal nonaction to a graduated path upon which simple technical meditations can hie us on our way. But as his compassionate concern allows in the root text, "Different strokes for different folks". It would appear that the root text was the original text and that the commentary was the later addition, rather than that the root text was a mnemonic summary of the original longer text, which is sometimes the case. Some of the cantos are short and show a unitary theme throughout; others are much longer and the divisions indicated in the commentary are not immediately evident as changing themes in the original treatise. Indeed the topics treated by the commentary are sometimes difficult to locate in the original as if the commentator were attempting to put a round theme into a square context.

Then to the matter of secrecy: Dzogchen is considered secret in the Nyingma tradition that carries it. It is deemed so in various ways. Firstly, Dzogchen is secret insofar as some minds are incapable intellectually of understanding the topic or the vocabulary or grammar in the Tibetan or in any other language. Secondly, it is secret insofar as many people may understand the topic and the syntax but cannot grasp the meaning of Dzogchen, in the same way that many educated people in the West cannot comprehend a textbook of advanced mathematics. Thirdly, it is secret because the meaning may be grasped intellectually but because what is described is beyond that mind to comprehend in terms of its own past or potential experience, the meaning is not retained, no advantage accrues and the secret remains locked. In these three ways the text is self-secret.

It is also deemed secret in that some lamas conceal the subject matter of Dzogchen texts like *The Treasury of the Dharmadhatu* from certain groups of people. Lamas of the tradition may wish to keep the most privileged instruction in their own family or monastic lineage for both selfish personal or altruistic religious reasons or for both. Thus certain qualifications are required of recipients before the transmission can be conveyed or the book can be read. The lineage holders thereby maintain control of the literature and practice. Magical incantations, malediction or curses attached to such works drive fear into the hearts of potentially duplicitous readers or practitioners. Notations added to the texts threaten dire consequences if the samayas (commitments) laid upon the initiates are broken.

Within the practice-lineage, one practical reason for keeping the text secret is to prevent general conceptual information about the practices that the text contains prejudicing the yogin's intellect against personalized meditation instruction transmitted at a later, propitious moment. In other words, an empty, nonconceptual mind is preferred in the recipient of Dzogchen meditation instruction. Mere information about the precepts obstructs transmission. Similarly, the texts are kept from some insiders because it is thought that damage could be done either to their minds or to their process in attainment of nirvana. In recent years, these seminal Dzogchen texts were kept from westerners for one or more of these reasons. A lama may have thought, for instance, that Westerners were simply incapable of understanding the texts, a conception based upon the common Chinese cultural prejudice that all Europeans were barbarians or morons or both. Another reservation was provided by the lama's fear that the material would be stolen and published elsewhere for uncontrolled public consumption. Perhaps it was to be misused, where misuse constituted any purpose other than the support of personal, guided meditation in the conventional manner. Unfortunately this reservation was indeed sometimes proven valid by western researchers who took "secret" instruction under the pretense of Buddhist commitment, but in search of fame and fortune in the western academy published the material without regard for the lamas' sensibility. Likewise, librarians or obsessive collectors of Tibetan texts would extract books from lamas under false pretenses. Some traditionalist lamas object to their sacred texts being taken and processed in secular western media, their holy dharma disrespected thereby, in much the same way that some Muslims believe their sacred Koran should be held only in the hands of believers.

An important historical reason why secrecy was maintained lies in the relationship between the Nyingma and the yellow hat school. While quite distinct from the sudden school of Chinese Ch'an (or Japanese Zen), Dzogchen was identified with it by the right wing gradualists in the early debate between scholars of the Indian Madhayamika school and those of the Tibetan, Chinese-influenced Dzogchen. This misconception was sustained by the Kadampa school and later by their Gelukpa successors. This identification of Dzogchen with the apostasy of the "sudden" school, which began at the Council of Lhasa in the eighth century, condemned the Nyingma school, which carried the Dzogchen teaching, to a peripheral political status. In the eighteenth century, insupportable pressure from the Gelukpas at the height of their political and military power in Lhasa pressured the principal Nyingma lama of the time, the great terton Gyurme Dorje at Mindroling, the principal seat of the Nyingma in Central Tibet, into an accord with the Gelukpas. Whatever the stated, "public", announcement of the Fifth Dalai Lama's accord with Gyurme Dorje, the actual effect was to bury radical Dzogchen deeply within a newly asserted Nyingma monastic hegemony. Therein it was available only to the elite tulkus and very bright khenpos at the end of a long and arduous Buddhist cultural education. The ancient tradition of lay lamas living in village gompas or in secular housing with large shrines was attenuated, and along with it the secular ngakpa tradition. In Kham, Eastern Tibet, which thereafter became the mainspring of dharmic activity and has remained so, the great families tended to have a parallel lineage of father-to-son transmission in the great gompas through the convention of tulku succession. The virulent criticism and even persecution that the Nyingma Dzogchen practitioners were subjected to by the Gelukpas, however, was ample reason to keep the teaching secret, in spite of successive Dalai Lamas' covert practice of Dzogchen. The present Dalai Lama, Tenzin Gyatso, has attempted to give new status and acceptability to Dzogchen in the face of unprecedented refusal and outright rejection from certain Geluk schools.

Longchen Rabjampa (1308 - 1364)

Longchenpa was born in the heart of Tibet in the rich and fertile valley of Dra in Yoru, on the southern side of the Tsangpo. Apart from the years of his exile to Bumthang in Bhutan, he was to spend his life in Central Tibet. His father was the village priest of Todrong descended from an eminent line of married Nyingma lamas that traced their ancestry back to the family of Gyelwa Chokyang, one of Padma Sambhava's twenty-five disciples. Both his father and grandfather were yogin adepts. A precocious boy, he could read and write by the age of five. His early practice focused on the eight Nyingma buddha-deities but he also studied and memorized vinaya and prajnaparamita texts. At the age of twelve, he was ordained as a novice at Samye and in his adolescence he studied the *Chakrasamvara-tantra* and the six doctrines of Vajravarahi, the Path and Fruit (lamdre) system of the Sakyas, and the Kalachakra, amongst others.

At the age of nineteen he was admitted to the Kadampa academy-cum-seminary at Sangphu in the Kyichu valley, which was then Sakya dominated and provided the finest foundation of scholarship in Tibet. The Nyingma tantras and transmissions were his primary concern but also, in particular, he studied the Kagyu tradition under the Dzogchen master the third Karmapa Rangjung Dorje, and the Sakya tradition under Lama Dampa Sonam Gyeltsen. He was nonsectarian, investigating all contemporary schools. At the end of his study at Sangphu, he received the title Rabjampa.

He left Sangphu disenchanted by the academic institution with its political in-fighting and scholarly narrow-mindedness and took to the contemplative life of a homeless yogin that he was to practice for the rest of his life. Early on, during a dark retreat in Gyama, he had a vision of a sixteen-year-old dakini protectress that heralded a visionary life dominated by the dakinis wherein they guided him, blessed him and taught him.

In 1336, at the age of twenty-eight, he met Rigzin Kumaraja (1266-1343), a knowledge-bearer yogin who travelled around Central Tibet teaching a small coterie of close disciples. Longchenpa followed him for a number of years suffering deep privation, living on herbs, with only a blanket to keep him warm. Kumaraja, a Karma Kagyu yogin, the disciple of the Dzogchen master Melong Dorje and also an initiate of Bonpo Dzogchen, became Longchenpa's Dzogchen guru and from him received the entire corpus of Dzogchen initiation, transmission and instruction. Kumaraja eventually appointed him his lineal successor.

In his thirty-first year, Longchenpa began to teach the Dzogchen Nyingtik, at Nyiphu Shuksep, not far from Sangphu. That same year, Wozer Gocha discovered the Khandro Nyingtik and gave it to Longchenpa to examine. The following year while giving initiation to eight yogis and yoginis at Gangri Tokar, close to Shuksep, the ganachakra feast became an actual wild communion of participants with dakinis and protectors in which the precept "mind free from meditation is the bliss" became an actual experience. At this ganachakra Longchenpa received final confirmations and injunctions from Vajravarahi herself specifying the Vimala Nyingtik and Khandro Nyingtik as his mode of practice and teaching. Later in the same month, Padma Sambhava himself accompanied by his retinue appeared from the Southwest and was seen to vanish into Longchenpa. That night while Longchenpa making the inner offering, Padma Sambhava appeared with Vimalamitra on his right and Vajravarahi on his left with dakinis blowing thighbone trumpets in front while behind was a crowd of yogins and dakinis singing and dancing. During both these visionary experiences, the Dakini Vajravarahi clarified his mind and confirmed her constant presence.

Soon after, Longchenpa started writing, and his output was so immense that it beggars belief. Was he the editor of his many disciples' works or their works based on his oral teaching? Did later collectors and editors of his work include the tomes of the many great Dzogchen yogis that flourished at that time? He certainly wrote under different names, so many that a complete inventory has not been made. *The Seven Treasuries* were his greatest works, and *The Treasury of the Dharmadhatu* was the greatest of the seven.

In his forties, he had become an eminent hermit, his principal hermitage Gangri Tokar, where he did most of his writing. But he had interests outside his prose composition, *kavya* poetry and revelations of treasure. In 1349, he restored the ancient Zhai Lhakhang temple and re-erected its inscribed pillars. He rebuilt the stupa of Shantarakshita on Hepori and conserved the abbot's skull. In his latter years, he sired three children by different women, and one of his sons, Chodak Zangpo, wrote a biography of his father. He became a preceptor of the Drigungpas, the old power of Central Tibet, and incurred the wrath of Situ Changchub Gyeltsen, the chief of the rising Kagyu power. After he miraculously escaped an assassination attempt, in 1354 he exiled himself to Bumthang in Bhutan. He later returned to Central Tibet and was reconciled with Situ, but he died soon after in Chimphu in 1364 at the age of 56.

Acknowledgements

I acknowledge the crucial debt I owe to all those near and far, Christian and Buddhist, Beatnik and Hippy, Indian and Tibetan, Guru and Dakini, who have shown me the nature of mind. I would like to thank Jeremiah and Catherine Weser and Mimi Church for their assistance in preparation of this manuscript.

Prologue

Introductory

The luminous mind, its clear light and its spontaneity, are the topics of this poem, and this reality is all and always only known in the now, beyond categories of past, present and future. We can never know anything except in the now. Direct perception provides the only knowledge worthy of the name. The now is the space of direct and immediate experience and that space is called "the matrix of the now". Everything that is known is known in the matrix of the now. This knowledge includes Dzogchen reality and samsara and nirvana, all of which is experienced as the now. In successive cantos, Longchenpa describes the now as spaciousness, and then as buddhafields, and then as luminous mind. The now is evoked in and as nonstriving and noncausality, and in and as inclusivity and spontaneity, and in and as nonduality. The now is shown as resolution and as guru-vision, as purity and release, and finally the here and now is revealed as buddha.

The space of the now is called "the matrix" (Tib: *klong*) and this word will appear hundreds of times in Longchenpa's poem. Everything occurs in the matrix of the now. Everything we know we cognize in the matrix of the now. Nothing neither exists nor does not exist outside the matrix of the now. The matrix of the now is another way of saying our "being". In his prologue Longchenpa identifies cognition in the matrix of the now as the "apex perspective", the "vajra-heart" and "the natural state of being". It is the "clear light"; it is "spontaneity". It is present without action or effort. It is, in the conventional phrase, "a vast expanse".

Direct experience of the here and now is represented anthropomorphically as the Buddha Kuntuzangpo, Samantabhadra, the All-Good Buddha. Merely by acknowledging him, paying homage to him, as the spontaneity of the clear light of the luminous mind, we receive the Dzogchen transmission of *Spaciousness*. Thus, the transmission is received by acknowledgement of the now as the spaciousness of mind's natural disposition. This is the all-good reality that Longchenpa evokes in this prologue and in the following thirteen cantos.

PROLOGUE

Homage to Glorious Kuntuzangpo, Sri Samantabhadra,
Homage to the All-Good Buddha.

Homage to pristine spontaneity, the clear light of luminous mind,
The amazing reality of this fantastic universe,
A treasury of self-sprung awareness in the now,
And the source of everything, samsara and nirvana.
Homage to that motionless space of simplicity.

This matrix of the apex approach, the peak orbited by sun and moon,
This matrix of the vajra-heart, the clear light of spontaneity,
This matrix is naturally disposed without effort or practice:
Listen while I describe this awesome investiture of the now.

Canto One: Spaciousness

Introductory

Spaciousness is the title of this poem and the first canto treats spaciousness. If this text is an experiential introduction to the nature of mind, it points repeatedly at spaciousness. If the true nature of all things – reality – is to be characterized at all, then spaciousness is the word that best fits the experience. So, in this first canto, the Dzogchen adept makes his radical experience absolutely clear: reality is the matrix of the spaciousness in which all appearances arise but never become anything else than the sameness that is their source. In Mahayana Buddhist jargon, everything arises in emptiness and never ceases to be emptiness, so emptiness is all we have. In Dzogchen parlance, spaciousness is like emptiness, and in the Dzogchen way of seeing things, since emptiness is never separate from form, so it is with spaciousness. Everything is total spaciousness and nothing else; but everything arises in spaciousness and although all the phenomena that "everything" denominates can never crystallize and be labeled as concrete things, they cannot be denied. They are best described as "apparition" or "illusion". Our intellect – ordinary relative mind – tends to turn those airy, amorphous forms into concrete things – to reify them. Not only that, but it locates them in time, so that over a succession of moments they may appear to be in motion and therefore ephemeral in their constant change. In reality, in the vast matrix of the now, in a timeless moment, everything is unmoving, and thus the all-pervasive expanse of self-aware spaciousness is said to be immutable.

The primary implication of this experiential intimation of reality is the crucial realization that samsara and nirvana are nothing other than their intrinsic spaciousness. No distinction can exist, actually, between appearance and emptiness, between what we perceive and its absence.

In this Longchenpa's Dzogchen exposition, it is useful to remember that for Tibetan Buddhists "existence" implies a substantial core – a self, an *ens*, a soul, an *atman* – that subsists in human beings, at least from birth to death. For seemingly external appearances, "existence" implies something like an essential discrete particle that cannot be destroyed or divided. Of course, no such thing "exists", either in the bodymind or in external entities. Thus, since there is no "existence", what we perceive is all we can get and there is no distinction between perceiving something and perceiving nothing at all. It is all illusion, and that is the beginning of the Dzogchen view.

It is not enough to compute the absence of any substantial existence deductively; it is imperative that we realize it existentially. This realization is not to be instilled as an alternative to the belief in existence inside the skin or outside it; on the contrary, such understanding arises only when we let go of all beliefs whatsoever, including belief in God, gods, the Buddha and the possibility of attaining any spiritual goal such as nirvana. Such deconstruction may be effected initially – perhaps when we first approach philosophical Buddhism – by the intellect, but very soon it becomes clear that the intellect can only place us at the door of understanding and that existential realization is the product of an intuitive faculty that lies within consciousness itself. The experience that this intuitive faculty provides is what Longchenpa expresses in this poem.

It appears that Longchenpa is going to follow the conventional pyramidal structure of such texts, starting at an apex, which is like the vajra-heart itself, the all-inclusive totality, the heart essence, and fanning out in subsequent cantos to describe its increasingly elaborate ramifications. Not so. Each canto maintains the same intensity and holistic integrity; each canto is a wide open door into the nature of mind; each canto describes a separate label of ultimacy, a label of the luminous mind of spontaneity that is the now, and the first and foremost of those labels is "spaciousness".

SPACIOUSNESS

"Samsara and nirvana never stir from their intrinsic spaciousness."

Everything arises in the vast matrix of spontaneity
And spontaneity is the ground of everything,
But empty in essence, never crystallizing,
The ground is nothing although it appears as everything.
Samsara and nirvana arise as spontaneity in the trikaya[1] matrix,
Yet they can never stir from their intrinsic spaciousness,
For such are the blissful fields of reality.

The nature of mind is an unchanging, skylike supermatrix,
A matrix of variable display, compassionate magical emanation –
Everything is ornamentation of spaciousness, and nothing else.
It is the creativity of luminous mind, pulsating outward and inward,
Being nothing at all, yet appearing as everything whatsoever,
And it paints magnificent, amazing, magical emanation.

Outside and inside, and the material and spiritual dimensions,
Are ornaments of spaciousness arising as the wheel of sublime form;
All sounds and speech, everything that vibrates,
Are ornaments of spaciousness arising in essence as sublime vibration;
All movement of thought, and all inconceivable nonthought,
Are ornaments of spaciousness arising as the wheel of sublime mind.

The six kinds of mythic beings,[2] moreover, with four types of birth,[3]
Can never stray an iota from the spaciousness of their reality,
And the six fields[4] of dualistic sense perception of the universe,
Appearing in their own spaciousness, like magical illusion, do not
    truly exist;
Baseless, vividly apparent, yet empty in the now, supremely spacious,
With natural clarity, they appear as decoration of their intrinsic
    spaciousness.

No matter what the perception arising in this vast spaciousness,
In its unremitting sameness it is the dharmakaya of luminous mind;
Disposed in the now, empty in itself, unchanging, unsublimating,

As self-sprung awareness in the now, reality itself,
Effortlessly, passively, it is part of the one blissful matrix.

In its unchanging intrinsic clarity it is sambhogakaya,
And however is manifests it is spontaneity,
Uncontrived and unalloyed in its unremitting sameness.

Whatever the shape of the distinct, multifarious display,
Its reality is self-sprung emanation, magical projection,
And it never strays from the nonaction of the All-Good.

In the fail-safe luminous mind
The unfabricated trikaya is already perfected;
Not stirring from spaciousness, its spontaneity uncompromised,
The activity of buddha in buddhafields[5] is already perfected;
The matrix of sublime spontaneity dawns in the now,
Universal multiplicitous diversity[6] perfected in the now.

This field of unalterable, unsublimating spontaneity in the now,
This is the visible reality of intrinsic spaciousness,
Noncrystallizing knowledge arising to ornament that spaciousness;
Already arrived, nothing to do, without any practice,
Like the sun in the sky – that is an amazing, superb reality.

Here in this womb-like spaciousness, in the spontaneity of the now,
Samsara is all good and while nirvana is also good
In this all-good matrix, in the now, neither samsara nor nirvana exist.
Appearances are all good, and while emptiness is also all good
In this all-good matrix, in the now, neither appearance nor emptiness
    exist.
Life is all good, and while good and bad feelings are also all good
In this all-good matrix neither life nor feelings exist.
Self and other are both all good
And while acceptance and rejection are also all good
In this all-good matrix, no self and other, no affirmation or negation
    is possible.

In delusion we reify what is not truly existent and label it.
Why is it that we so readily affix attributes to samsara and nirvana,
When their nature is so dream-like, baseless and evanescent?

Everything is all good, magnificent spontaneity,
And delusion never having existed in the past,
Existing neither in the present nor the future,
"Life" is just a label, the paradox of being and nonbeing resolved.
No one has ever been deluded anywhere in the past,
No one is deluded now, and no one will be deluded in the future:
That is alpha-pure vision of past, present and future.[7]

When delusion is nonexistent, nondelusion cannot exist,
And, spontaneously in the now, pure presence is right here;
Since there never was release, is no release now, and never will be,
"Nirvana" is a mere label and no one has ever known liberation;
There can be no release because no confinement can exist in the now.
And pure like the sky, nothing can ever be restricted or localized:
That is alpha-pure vision of ultimate liberation.

In short, in the spontaneity of this vast womb-like spaciousness,
What seems to be samsara or nirvana is a display of creativity,
That at its very inception is neither samsara nor nirvana.
Further, no matter what dream arises in the creativity of sleep,
It is, in truth, an absence, a blissful rest in natural presence,
Smoothly spaced out in vast, unremitting sameness!

Canto Two: Buddhafields

Introductory

With realization of the awareness intrinsic to consciousness, all perception is described as decoration or adornment of its inherent spaciousness. But to say that the forms of perception are predicated upon that spaciousness is to invent spaciousness as a separate or distinct entity or substance, and in the previous canto that has been conclusively shown to be impossible. The mode of being as buddha and its awareness are an all-encompassing unity. Buddha is not separate from the field and the awareness is a self-aware field that includes buddha – thus "buddhafield". That is like saying that the buddhafield is aware of itself and that the person who is being aware is included therein without acknowledgement of a separate identity. It is like saying that all sentient beings are a part of a vast unitary panorama, sharing its sameness and its clear light and its awareness in the now.

The buddhafield manifests when the witness to an event is not separate from awareness, primal awareness, awareness in the now. Insofar as no witness raises its head, no objectivity pertains in the moment of the now. The now is the crucible of the event. So a buddhafield is not like a magical garden in a Persian legend where jeweline fruit are hanging from branches of gold on a tree growing out of a landscape of semi-precious stones. Rather, nothing is seen there but sameness, smoothness, an evenness of perception, as in an incipient perception, a perception before the intellect has categorized and labeled, filtered and projected. The level of integration implied here, the level of unity, is usefully likened to the level of pixelation on a computer screen. Behind the letters of the text, behind the lines and colors of the visuals, are the pixels. If the pixels are defocused then, instead of a field of white points, we see fields of spaciousness.

The text, or the visuals, are then not distinct from the pixelated field, from the spaciousness. But this is a mere simile for the unity of the dharmadhatu with the multifarious forms that arise within it, the unified field of the single maha-pixel, the one sole ultimate sphere. We should not think that buddhafields truly exist anywhere at all. They have no location; they are indeterminate and of uncertain being, like a peripatetic, homeless yogin. This canto mentions buddhafields only once and then only as a counterpoint to the six mythic realms of samsara and to assert that both buddhafields and samsaric realms have their ground in spaciousness. Buddhafields in the Dzogchen context are identical to the threefold trikaya reality, which comprises the three dimensions of being that are inherent in the natural disposition, the spaciousness of reality. We cannot attain buddhafields by design or by practice. We cannot get there by plan, intent or aspiration. Buddhafields do not truly exist, so how can we attain them? A buddhafield is a flash of the clear light of pure presence spontaneously illuminating a nanosecond of consciousness of one of the sensory fields that constitute the supermatrix of the here and now. It occurs in such a way as to make that instant of awareness a unitary experience of spaciousness where the form and the awareness are an inseparable, ineffable hit or blast of clarity. The buddhafield is an intimation of the form and the awareness as a unitary experience of spaciousness.

The six mythic realms of samsara are buddhafields. The realms of the gods, demons, human beings, hungry ghosts, animals and denizens of hell, founded in the spaciousness of the matrix of the now and thus pure in their own nature, are spontaneously assimilated to pure presence and cannot escape its unitary awareness, the primal awareness in the now. What were seen as projections of the intellect are now realized as self-envisioned illusory figments of mind, phantoms of delight. Deconstructed, reduced to mere color and shape in a pixelated ocean, the beings of the six realms and their environments are perceived as buddhafields.

Insofar as a buddhafield is a nondual experience of spaciousness, only one buddhafield is knowable, and that is beyond the intellect to comprehend and beyond differentiation and classification. So why in Dzogchen are there said to be an incalculable number of buddhafields, and why are innumerable buddhafields individually named in Vajrayana and Mahayana Buddhism? The incalculable number of buddhafields refers to the incalculable number of moments of temporal experience that may be recognized as timeless moments of experience of the dharmadhatu. The names that are given to some moments refer to buddha representing a particular color or mental function, a buddha-deity that represents an aspect of the totality (the physical, energetic or mental activity, or potential, for example). Or it may be the name of the bodhisattva that guards a sensory field, the buddha-consort that represents one of the great elements, or a buddha-dakini who represents a complementary aspect of buddha with which she consorts. But these buddhafields, like Amitabha's Dewachan, Kalachakra's Shambhala, Padma Sambhava's Copper-Colored Mountain and so on, are all conceptual images designed to provide inspiration or to act as a carrot to wave before the yogin-donkey's nose to urge him to strive harder along the long graduated path of progressive Buddhism. Alternatively, they may be poetic conceits contrived to amuse and delight those of "little brain" by visionary adepts who walk the pathless path.

BUDDHAFIELDS

"Our fields of perception are buddhafields."

The spaciousness that is pristine spontaneity
Pervades everything, joining outside and inside;
It has no boundaries, top or bottom, and is beyond direction.
As pure presence, it is clear like the sky, nonspatial, nondual;
As the vast matrix itself, it is beyond pulsating thought and image.

The magical illusion that emanates within this unborn spaciousness,
Quite indeterminate, without any definition whatsoever,
Cannot be denominated as something for it has no substance or
    attribute.
Insofar as its skylike nature fills space-time,
It is unborn spontaneity -- no before or after, no beginning or end.

The nature of all samsara and nirvana is this luminous mind,
Unmanifest, unproduced, indeterminate spontaneity,
Coming from nowhere and going nowhere;
The matrix of luminous mind indicates neither past nor future,
For it is unvarying in its all-pervasive uniformity.

Reality, just as it is, without beginning, middle or end,
An all-pervasive smoothness, is skylike in nature:
Without either beginning or end, it supersedes linear time;
Without origination or cessation, it can have neither substance nor
    attribute;
It is invariable, so it cannot be denominated as any "thing";
It cannot be induced or practiced, so nothing is to be done;
And without mass or volume, it is the ground of suchness.

Unimageable and unassailable, it is the matrix of sameness;
Since sameness is the reality of all things,
Everything necessarily rests in the matrix of sameness;
This luminous mind is a singularity in which all is equal,
And since its all-pervasive smoothness is like unmanifest space,
Within that gamut of sameness, there can be no intervention.

This fortress of nontemporal spontaneity, all-pervasive,
This fortress of the vast matrix of the now, without top, bottom or
    middle,
This fortress of the unborn dharmakaya, impartially all-accommodating,
This fortress of the precious secret that is unchanging spontaneity –
This fortress of the now, the entire galaxy, samsara and nirvana,
This is the totality, the single denominator.

Upon a zero-dimensional, all-pervasive foundation,
Stands the palace of luminous mind, samsara and nirvana identical;
At its marvelously high pinnacle is the vast matrix of reality,
The center of an uncreated omni-dimensional panorama,
A wide-open doorway to freedom from graduated endeavor.

Within that palace arrayed with spontaneously amassed wealth,
The king Self-Sprung Awareness takes his throne;
His pulsating projections, emanations of his pristine awareness,
Serve as ministers who govern his domain;
The holy queen Innate Meditative Absorption attends
With Spontaneous Guru-Vision, her offspring, and her servants,
All centered in the pure pleasure matrix of intrinsic, nonconceptual
    clarity.

Within that still, ineffable plenum,
The king masters all manifest and potential appearances,
And the immense dominion of vast spaciousness is his.

Living in that land, everything is dharmakaya:
Never straying from our unitary self-sprung awareness in the now,
Seizing the uncreated now, beyond striving and practice,
Encompassed by the one sole sphere that has no hard edges,
Just as we are, we are centered in that undifferentiated, all-inclusive
  matrix.

Since the six mythic realms and even the buddhafields
Shine nowhere but in that skylike reality,
In that inherently clear luminous mind they are of one taste,
And samsara and nirvana are naturally assimilated to pure presence.

In this treasury of existential spaciousness, the universal source,
Nirvana, unsought, is the constant spontaneity of the now;
So given the dharmakaya as unchanging, nonreferential, all-investing,
Internal and external visions, all life forms, are the sambhogakaya
And the nirmanakaya is like naturally occurring reflection.
So all experience necessarily ornamenting the three kayas,
It is all empty physical, energetic and mental display,
And the countless buddhafields, likewise, without exception,
All arise from the same source, the nature of mind, the trikaya matrix.

The contents of samsara, the six realms and their inhabitants,
Also, surely, are mere reflections within intrinsic spaciousness;
All the phantasmagoria of life and death, pleasure and pain,
Like apparitional show, abound in the matrix of mind in itself;
Apparent, yet insubstantial and hence truly nonexistent,
It occurs through adventitious circumstance,
Like moisture condensing as clouds;
Neither existent nor nonexistent, beyond determinate extremes,
It is all included in the one sole sphere where nothing is elaborated.

The nature of mind, the essential luminous mind,
Pure like the sky, free of birth and death, pleasure and pain,
Unaffected by materiality, is indifferent to samsara and nirvana;

It cannot be indicated as some "thing" for it is a vast skylike matrix;
Unchanging and incapable of sublimation, it is unalloyed spontaneity;
Buddha lies in the vajra-heart that is clear light,
Where everything is fields of self-sprung bliss,
Everything the unremitting sameness of that supreme light.

Canto Three: The Simile for Luminous Mind

Introductory

If we have pickled our minds in Mahayana scripture or commentary at some time in our lives, then we probably need to update our associations with bodhi-mind, bodhichitta and indeed bodhi-tree and bodhi-this and bodhi-that. Regarding reality – which means the nondual reality of Dzogchen – bodhi is a word that evokes the very nature of mind as experienced in the nontemporal, nonspatial discrete slice of perception of the now. From the point of view of the urban yogi, the one who is perceiving, the one who is part of the buddhafield, all experience is known as luminous mind, bodhi-mind, bodhichitta, the here and now. Bodhichitta was originally used in Mahayana Buddhism to designate the Buddha's mind; it was not meant in the Dzogchen sense of experience here and now, but as the enlightened mind that the bodhisattva sought to accomplish through virtuous and thought-free activity. It became the keyword in the luminous mind series of atiyoga precepts and as the first and basic perspective on Dzogchen. Although luminous mind is presented already in the third canto, it should be recalled that Longchenpa has gone beyond the threefold atiyoga classification (mind, matrix and secret precept) in his presentation of the vajra-heart.

The nature of luminous bodhi-mind is often described as "timeless", and the concept of "timeless mind" should evoke a state that is beyond the temporal parameters of past, present and future. But the danger is that in our minds conditioned in this post-Christian era "timeless" is understood as eternal, a constant without beginning or end, and remaining caught in a morass of concepts we risk falling into the pit of eternalism. This quicksand of the intellect menaces all of us who, just now, in the latter twentieth century, shook off the naïve Christian assumptions about the nature of being and the nature of mind. The antidote to both the intellectual malaise and the existential indifference that characterizes contemporary attitudes is a strengthening of the sense of the now, and that fortitude is supplied by the pointing out of the nature of mind, which is always an introduction to awareness in the now.

This exposition of the vajra-heart's core remains jammed in the intellect unless we can utilize the intellect to deconstruct – experientially through nonmeditation, not intellectually with discursive thought – the concepts that comprise it, and set free what phrases such as "intrinsic spaciousness", "unremitting sameness", and first and foremost "spontaneity" are pointing at. "Timeless", "primordial", "original" and 'pristine" are all synonyms of alpha-pure, the keyword that qualifies the trekcho modality, and the only home of alpha-purity is the here-and-now, which is always with us, constantly pushing the natural state of being into the light of day, never to be denied, inescapable, the crucible of all our knowing.

The simile of the holographic pixel was outside Longchenpa's cultural frame – it is well within ours. While "the ultimate sphere", "the one sole sphere" of Dzogchen, the "*thig-le*" of tantra-yoga and anuyoga, and the "cosmic egg" of new age metaphysics, does talk to us, the single cell of a hologram in which the entire hologram is contained, the microcosm in which the macrocosm is contained, whereby macrocosm and microcosm are equalized, is a more powerful image. An image that is even closer to home, evident to a child (or a geriatric) cell-phone user, is the invisible pixel of the LCD screen, or the subliminal pixel of a photographic print. Although this pixel does not contain the propensity to regenerate the whole from the part, a single pixel itself, identical in nature to every other pixel in the square inch of screen or print, nevertheless carries a separate and unique piece of information that makes the pixel itself unique. The word "pixel", therefore, is an excellent potential equivalent of the word *thig-le* (Tibetan) and *bindu* (Sanskrit) as used in Dzogchen and an excellent simile for luminous mind, enlightened mind, the nature of mind – for reality itself.

THE SIMILE FOR LUMINOUS MIND

"Everything comes together in luminous mind."

Since luminous mind excludes nothing whatsoever,
So all experience is of the nature of luminous mind.

The simile for luminous mind is "skylike".
Because that mind has no cause and cannot be objectified
It has no location, it is ineffable and beyond ideation,
So "the spaciousness of the sky" is an apt metaphor.
If the metaphor denotes nothing specific,
How could it evoke anything definite?
Understand that the sky is a metaphor for natural purity.

What is evoked is the skylike intrinsic presence of luminous mind,
Incapable of verbalization, defying illustration and description;
Such is the vast matrix of intrinsic clarity, motionless clear light,
Uncontrived spontaneity without status or dimension –
It is the dharmakaya, the wide-open center of the luminous heart.

It is evinced by whatever arises as creativity,
At its point of inception without base or creator;
What does arise, being mere label,
Vanishes into spaciousness when identified.
Assimilated into undifferentiated virginal sameness,
Free of perceptual duality, it is the matrix of spaced-out smoothness.

*

This zero-dimensional reality of self-sprung awareness in the now,
Revealed by analogy – well-defined similitude, evocation and evidence,
The very essence denoted by these three beautiful sky-bolts,[8]
Assimilates everything without differentiation or exclusion.
In the womb-like space of this vast expanse of equality,
In the now, everything is always the same,
Without temporal or qualitative distinction:[9]
That is the vision of Samantabhadra Vajrasattva.

Luminous mind is like the solar nucleus:
Its nature is clear light, forever uncompounded;
Nothing can veil its translucent spontaneity,
And as unthought reality, elaborate variation is impossible.

The dharmakaya as emptiness, the sambhogakaya as clarity
And the nirmanakaya as radiance are three kayas,
Yet they can never be united or separated,
And since in the now their potential is wrought in spontaneity,
Darkening flaws and faults cannot veil them;
They are identical in their changelessness and timelessness,
Identical in their saturation of buddhas and sentient beings alike,
Identical as "self-sprung luminous mind".

The creativity of that luminous mind occurs as any damn thing,
As thought or nonthought,[10] as manifestation or potential,
As diverse and various as living beings' perceptions!

Things appear but they never crystallize:
Everything is like mirage, dream, echo,
Like apparition, reflection in water and castles in the sky.
Like hallucination, things are clearly apparent, but do not truly exist.
Know all experience as rootless and baseless, mere adventitious
    appearance,
Just ephemeral occurrence, circumstantial and contingent.

In the spontaneous nature of luminous mind,
The display noncrystallizing, samsara and nirvana emanate magically,
To be assimilated simultaneously into its spaciousness:
Know that display does not stray from its original natural perfection.

Here and now everything lies within the scope of luminous mind:
Perfect in its oneness, perfect in its all-inclusiveness,
Everything perfect in its natural, uncontrived reality,
As perfection, it is self-sprung awareness in the now.

Since luminous mind is neither visible nor invisible,
Neither outer nor inner, samsara nor nirvana can exist concretely,

Yet by virtue of its dynamic creativity, the myriad display,
The material and spiritual dimensions, samsara and nirvana, shine out.

Forms that at their very inception are essentially empty,
Unborn but appearing to be born,
Appear, yet nothing whatsoever has been created;
Nothing crystallizes, although it may appear to do so,
And that noncrystallizing illusion is the form of emptiness.
Even in its apparent stability, nothing real subsists,
For groundless and changeless whatever appears,
And however it appears, it can never be substantiated,
And so it is labeled simply "insubstantial".

Since appearances appear by themselves in creativity,
They are said, symbolically, to be "synchronicitous";
Arising in creativity, at the very moment of inception
No arising or nonarising can be said to occur, no time or space,
So "creativity" is a mere symbol-word designating nothing;
Since nothing neither alters nor sublimates,
How can it move an iota out of luminous mind?

Canto Four: Luminous Mind

Introductory

Physicists propose these days that constituents of the subatomic realm can be conceived as either waves or particles and that according to the perspective chosen by the perceiver, the reality remaining unchanged, particles act according to their preconceived nature. Likewise, in our everyday lives we are what we think we are. If we believe that we are separate entities, islands or bubbles of discrete being, separate from both material and spiritual environments, then we may best describe our experience in terms of the six mystic realms of samsara or in the terms of some similar analytic psychological frame. Perhaps we should add a codicil admitting that escape from the prison represented by any such frame is a distinct possibility – and that such escape could be called "nirvana". If on the other hand we believe that nothing substantial exists anywhere and so-called sensorial reality is no more than a commonly held delusion and that the nature of mind, buddha-mind, is inherent in every moment of consciousness, then we are setting ourselves up for experience of the great perfection. The concepts themselves, the belief system, will not actually induce experience of reality, because concepts are all the same in their status as display of the creativity of luminous mind. Yet insofar as Dzogchen is a statement of the natural state of being, intellectual acceptance of it allows the possibility of recognition of it – the words are doorways into the reality.

"Bodhi" in radical Dzogchen can be translated as "high", so that bodhichitta is "high-mind", with its connotations of high-mindedness and the state of mind that is awakened to its unbounded potential, infused with a spirit of unbridled compassion and a sense of infinite spontaneous accomplishment. "Bodhichitta" is often translated as awakened mind, but awakening implies a temporal process of raising the adept from a state of sleep and ignorance. The radical Dzogchen view insists that we have always been awake but that we have simply failed to recognize it. The sun is still shining, even though clouds veil it. The difference in these perspectives may appear slight; but every undermining leverage that we can apply to the intellect may assist us in sustaining our identity with the nature of mind.

With emphasis upon awareness and the view and meditation rather than cause and result, Dzogchen exposition has a tendency to diminish the connotation of compassion that bodhi-mind brings with it due to its long sojourn in the bodhisattva realm. "Compassion" in Dzogchen implies the four boundless states of mind: loving kindness, sympathetic joy, compassionate response and equanimity, because these four affections are the natural response to the suffering of beings that arise in its spontaneous awareness. Our own happiness manifests as these boundless qualities of bodhi-mind. "Compassion" is the six perfections of wisdom: generosity, morality, patience, perseverance, concentration and meditation. The nature of mind, bodhi-mind, naturally seeks the benefit of both oneself and others and these activities of the bodhisattva arise spontaneously, without compulsion or effort, out of luminous mind. Finally, "compassion" is what is conducive to the enlightenment of all beings and insofar as the means and the keys to that ultimate recognition are beyond intellectual comprehension, there is no movement of body, speech or mind that is excluded from possible induction of that benefit.

THE NATURE OF LUMINOUS MIND

"Luminous mind is all-inclusive."

Luminous mind is not appearance – it goes beyond appearance;
It is not simply emptiness – it goes beyond emptiness;
It is not truly existent – it has no concrete attribute;
It is not nonexistent – it pervades all samsara and nirvana.
Neither "is" nor "is not", its unremitting sameness is pristine
    spaciousness,
And without root, base or substance, it is nonspatial and
    nontemporal.

Pure presence, unbreakable, is the luminous matrix;
Skylike spaciousness, unalterable and unchangeable, saturates the now;
As self-sprung awareness in the now, incommensurate in the now,
Unborn, unceasing, it is contained in the one sole sphere;
Indeterminate, all embracing, it is zero dimensional.

The vajra-heart's core, motionless, unremitting sameness,
All suffusing supreme spaciousness, neither doable nor undoable –
This is not a domain that can be described in words.
Insight welling up as the presence intrinsic in every field,
The adept, free of discursive elaboration, vocal and mental,
Convinced that every field of experience is ineffable,
Entertaining neither meditation nor any object of meditation,
Need not eliminate either depressed or elated thought.

In the reality of empowering being[11] in the now,
Where concepts of self and other do not govern us,
The three realms[12] in themselves are buddhafields of sameness.

The victors of all time are self-envisioned purity,
And everything indiscriminately partaking of that totality
Not an iota of anything is to be attained elsewhere.
All experience effulgent in the vast matrix of mind's nature,
There is not the slightest movement out of actual sameness.

Without inside or outside, without disturbing pulsation,[13]
Luminous mind as the source dispels the darkness of extremes
And without the need of doing anything precludes any deviation.

People's unrealized strobe-like perception in the mundane world
And awareness of sublime forms in the now that is pure buddha,
Both arise within the creativity of pure presence
As noncongealing display permeated by skylike spaciousness.
Insofar as there can be realization of that spaciousness, or its absence,
Realization affords the pure perception of blissful buddha,
While nonrealization delivers the ignorant dualistic propensities
That manifest multifariously, yet, still, never stray from spaciousness.
Luminous mind is the actual condition of everything,

And attributes uncrystallizing, no matter what their variation,
It is evident as the pure spaciousness of inherently clear reality,
Without sharpness or blur,[14] as unrestricted pure presence.

This self-sprung spacious matrix is translucent[15] awareness in the now,
It is the clear light unveiled, without any outside or inside;
Intrinsic presence is thus a marvelous mirror of mind,[16]
And intrinsic spaciousness is a precious wishfulfilling gem.
Since everything occurs naturally without any quest,
Self-sprung awareness in the now is the glorious source of fulfillment.

Whatever innumerable transcendent qualities can be divined,
All arise *out of* spaciousness *as* spaciousness
And all arise as sublime, noncrystallizing skillful means;
As unborn spaciousness everything is spontaneously perfected,
All material things transfigured by the emptiness of the luminous matrix,
The emptiness adorned by the intrinsic presence of the luminous matrix.

In luminous mind, in the now,
There is no duality of appearance and emptiness
And in that nondual detachment far-out magical illusion appears;
Unborn spaciousness, lacking any time frame,
Remains an immutable matrix, undivided and uncompounded;
And buddha of all time as awareness of pure presence,
A luminous matrix of intrinsic presence saturating dualistic perception,
Without inside or outside, reality is spacious spontaneity.

Canto Five: Noncausality and Nonstriving

Introductory

A line in Longchenpa's commentary strikes at the fulcrum of our ignorance: "We think that our awareness has been obscured and that we need to purify the obscurations and we think that we need to develop enlightened qualities." That line defines our confusion. When clouds cover the sun, we say, "The sun is not shining". The sun certainly is shining and never ceases to shine. Likewise, when we are fixated upon our ignorance our awareness is still always shining. Our ignorance also requires the light of awareness in order to be identified as ignorance; our pain requires the light of the mind to shine within it in order that we recognize our suffering. Thus it is an error in our apprehension that calls for cultivation of buddha-potential. Buddha-potential, like primal awareness, is always ever-present, and perceptible – if only we would stop trying to locate and cultivate it. It is present in fundamental nondual awareness; intellectual dualistic striving obscures it. If we can intuit the truth of this argument then that alone is sufficient to allow us to fall naturally disposed into nonmeditation and nonaction. This sophism may simply restate the old adage that a glass half full is always to be preferred over a glass half empty, but such an understanding is enough to turn the mind around in the deep seat of consciousness (*metanoia*) and focus upon its spacious awareness rather than its supposed ignorance and delusion. Thereby, we are perpetually reminded of our intuition of the nature of mind, which constitutes the first essential precept of the first human bearer of the lineage, Garab Dorje.

"Flow" and "continuum" and "continuity" are not terms we can apply to nondual experience in the zero dimension. Although "flow" is an excellent metaphor for an experience if we are truly immersed in it, every apparent distinction between the outside and inside having vanished, leaving us with an overwhelming impression of a unitary whole, it inevitably carries the connotation of space-time. Likewise, although "continuum" may well describe the mindstream experience of thought and sensory perception, it is a synonym of time. Looking from outside, in the frame of dualistic space-time, an obvious, self-evident continuity of the nondual experience of the subjective knower; but within the adept himself, he has no sense of time whatsoever. Thus, the notion of continuity is as foreign to nonduality as the idea of an infinite series of momentary events, even if those moments of experience are without extension in time. Perhaps the paradox of an endless stream of timeless slices of experience is the best way to express the nullification of space-time.

The expression "zero dimension" conveys the ambience of the place of absence of space-time, a nontemporal and nonspatial place. This is the ineffable reality of the natural state of being. It is the ground of being, the foundation of all appearances, which necessarily partake of the same reality. It is preeminently, though, self-sprung awareness, which is self-cognizant, timeless spontaneity. This nonduality is perhaps best expressed in the Tibetan medium of the painted scroll as a buddhafield or pure-land. In Dzogchen, all buddhafields and pure-lands are the same, but in Vajrayana the buddhafields are characterized by the different buddhas that populate them. Adi-buddha such as Kuntuzangpo, buddha-deities such as Vajra Kilaya, or nirmanakaya buddha such as Padma Sambhava, may dominate, and any of these buddhafields will probably show a threefold representation allowing the three dimensions of the nature of being as separate aspects of the zero dimension.

The intellect can be defined first as linguistic articulation, entailing a structure that expresses itself in terms of a subject and an object, I and you, outside and inside and a vast inventory of dualisms including pleasure and pain and good and bad and sticking on right and wrong. Such an agenda entails a three-dimensional extension of space and its ten directions. The assumption of causality linking one moment of its structure to another provides another intractable dimension, namely, time. In that way, space-time is a creation of the intellect and everything in space-time is, therefore, the creativity of the mind.

To the average Tibetan, dharma is the religious Vajrayana culture of the monasteries. For the committed follower of Guru Rinpoche, the root-guru of radical Dzogchen, dharma is the manifestation of his mind's nature. In other words, the forms of momentary experience take Buddhist cultural forms because the average Tibetan has been steeped in Vajrayana culture since birth, and immersed in meditation since his initiatory experience. Sitting down, he tells his beads, for example; taking a walk, he circumambulates the stupa; reading a book it is probably a scripture; painting a picture it is a painted scroll (thanka); evacuating his bowels he makes an offering to the hungry ghosts, and so on. In the West, our dharma is founded in Christian, Jewish or post-Judeo-Christian culture and regardless of the degree to which we have immersed ourselves in Tibetan and Buddhist tradition our dharma is still basically Western in fabric, texture and form. In this perspective, then, if all culturally specific aspects are leeched out of dharma, what remains? It is, surely, just bare experience separate from any formal modality; it is the infrastructure of our being, which is referred to as the trikaya, the three dimensions or modes of being.

For that reason, the word *dharma* is here translated as the nonspecific "experience". If dharma is understood as any specific type of Buddhist practice, then that practice is a temporal practice, clothing the naked reality of Kuntuzangpo. In this Dzogchen, Buddhist forms of dharma, culturally specific dharma, has the same ontological status as any religious Christian practice, for example, or any post-Christian cultural norm such as driving a car, watching a video or shopping. What Longchenpa is presenting in this work is something beyond cultural form or personal habitual activity of body speech or mind. He is pointing at the sun even though it hides behind clouds.

The most radical Dzogchen maintains that goal-oriented spiritual praxis with liberation from samsara as the target is not only futile but that if it exists it at all it eventually nullifies itself – if it is not already a habit we need not start to practice it. In a less radical but still quasi-progressive way of thinking, spiritual praxis is considered drone-like activity without ultimate benefit, which could, however, be engaged upon as culturally valid behavior entailing socially beneficial qualities. The latter-day progressive school believes that if the natural state is not realized here and now then spiritual exercises will hasten the day that the state of nonaction will be realized. In other words, if aspiration is strong enough, if practice is sufficiently rigorous, if love of the guru is all-embracing, causal factors may induce a noncausal or an acausal state, and that meditative technique may induce a nondual state. Not only that, but on the progressive path one believes that meditative technique may eventually produce a state closer to the natural disposition of being and that the serendipitous state of nonaction is therefore more likely to occur. Some kind of special action can, it is said, actually induce nonaction. While the nature of mind cannot be attained through any cause or condition, it is held that certain conditions may actually cause it. Of course, it may be that spiritual praxis eventually leads to recognition of its own futility, in which case progressive Dzogchen is validated. But such a path entails deceiving an initiate into belief that the promise of success in attaining the ideal goal implies failure of the overt technical method. Further, the length of a path to its destination where the momentum that drives a spiritual seeker is eventually entirely appropriated cannot be estimated – the path may last forever.

One word that we hesitate to use to describe the state of mind that has understood the noncausal and unmotivated nature of mind is "aimless". It is poor commentary upon Western, post-Christian culture that an aimless state should be understood as a state of mindlessness and that both "aimlessness" and "mindlessness" are used generally to describe an undesirable state. If we are without aim we have no goal and if we have no goal we are sitting in perfect contentment in much the same way as a fool, a buffoon, an idiot – yet such aimlessness in the mind of the adept allows a spontaneous responsiveness that is compassionate and fully connected. Aimlessness, taken literally, is a close synonym of both noncausality and nonstriving and can subsume them both. It is, of course, impossible to be free of causality without having abandoned striving, and vice-versa. Aimlessness places us in the unlocatable spaciousness that is the ground of being, where spontaneity emanates its magical illusion. Aimlessness could be the title of this canto.

Longchenpa evokes the tantric path to illustrate the ineffectiveness of its techniques in inducing the great perfection. The proven difficulties of grafting tantric lifestyles onto Christian or post-Christian social modalities in western society is a contemporary and thus perhaps a more telling commentary upon those techniques. If tantric technique will not travel across cultural borders, if the rigid parameters of western society do not allow the expression of the samaya commitment that demands that naked awareness take priority over social norms, whether such techniques are functional or not is irrelevant. The ascetic tantric lifestyle is on the wane in India and Nepal where until now it has thrived in a lax, nondiscriminative, social milieu; likewise, the ritual tantric method cannot sustain itself in a quasi-western urban society in Asia.

Nonstriving, Noncausality

"Going Beyond Striving and Causality."

In the nature of mind, the luminous mind,
There is no view or meditation and no disciplinary training,
No goal to achieve, no stages or paths to traverse,
No mandala to create, no recitation of mantra, no fulfillment stage,
No empowerment to receive and no samaya to protect.
In the pure reality that is the spontaneity of the now
We are free of progressive, goal-oriented practices.

Yet the nature of those practices is luminous mind,
For the sun is always shining in spaciousness
Notwithstanding the veiling, adventitious, cloud.

The ten goal-oriented techniques[17] are taught,
In response to creativity's chance delusion,
As antidotes for those captivated by gradual progress.
It is not taught to adepts with genuine experience,
To those knowing the reality of atiyoga's vajra-heart.

To draw goal-oriented people striving on a graduated path
Towards the pristine spaciousness of reality,
The disciples', hermits' and bodhisattvas' approaches,[18]
The three lower vehicles, are taught in succession;
The kriya-tantra, upa-tantra and yoga-tantra approaches,
The three median vehicles, automatically follow.

And finally mahayoga, anuyoga and atiyoga,
The three higher approaches, are immanently evident;
Through the door of the progressive causal approaches
Fortunate beings are brought to threefold luminosity.[19]

The ultimacy of all approaches, however, is the vajra-heart,
That marvelous, sublime secret that all do share,
The apex that is unchanging, supreme clear light,
Celebrated as the revelation of the luminous heart.

Gradualists with discriminating, moral endeavor
Try to extinguish propensities manifesting as mind and mental events
That already, naturally, arise as a shining creative display:
They aspire to purify the mind that is already pristine awareness.

The supreme view makes no call upon discriminating endeavor,
For in reality direct encounter with the essence is inescapable –
Self-sprung awareness is the nature of luminous mind.
It is unnecessary desperately to search for it far afield.
Simply stay in yourself. You will find it nowhere else.

We know that reality itself, like the sun,
Stays forever in its natural state of all-embracing clear light;
Believing in their attempt to illuminate darkness
Others try to imitate the illuminating primordial sun:
The causal view is quite different from the supreme view.

Today some dinosaurs, taking pride in their atiyoga,
Believe sophisticated thought to be luminous mind.
Such fools are lost in a dark pit,
Self-exiled from the natural great perfection.
Ignorant of the creativity and the display of luminous mind,
How is it possible that they can know the luminous mind?

Here, we know that the alpha-pure luminous mind,
The true reality that is ultimate spaciousness,
Beyond thought and speech, is perfect insight;
We know it as inherently unmoving, intrinsic clear light,

In the now, free of all discursive elaboration.
It is what we mean by "essence", analogous to the solar nucleus;
Its creativity is noncrystallizing, unceasing pure presence,
Transparent and unlimited, free of conceptual and critical thought,
Shining with constant clarity, free of dualistic perception.

Creativity's pure presence entails intellectual functions,
Including dualistic perception and its manifold propensities:
The five sense objects, reifications of objects in a nonexistent field,
And the five afflictive emotions,[20] affects of a self that has no identity,
And all the delusory perceptions of outer universe and inner being –
If we fail to realize that delusory samsara, also, emerges from creativity,
In error we are caught in reified perceptual appearances.

With the realization that the supermatrix of reality
Comes from nowhere, goes nowhere, and stays nowhere,
"The vision of the total liberation of the three realms,"
The transmission of Ati, the spontaneity of the vajra-heart,
Arises in the matrix of the magnificent vastness of the All-Good.

Within the essence of immaculate luminous mind
There is nothing to see and no act of seeing,
Nothing to look at and no one to look,
No mind to meditate and nothing to meditate upon:
Because the conception and the act are one in spontaneity,
Not even a hint of a goal, nor rumor of a destination, occurs.

Because an indeterminate dharma has no structure,
There can never be a path to a goal.
Because the clear light is already a nondual sphere,
No mandala need be visualized by pulsating thought,
No mantra, no recitation, no empowerment, no samaya,
And no gradual dissolution in the fulfillment stage.
Immaculate buddha in buddhafields, already present in the now,
Cannot be created by causal concatenation.
If complex causality reigns, self-sprung awareness is precluded,
For what is compounded is subject to destruction
And how can that be called "simple spontaneity"?

So, in the nature of ultimate spaciousness,
Beyond causality, tantra's ten techniques are redundant;
Know that the genuine nature of mind, unmotivated,
Defuses all proliferating critical discursive thought.

Canto Six: Inclusivity

Introductory

One of the great beauties of Dzogchen is the stupidity that is all good, another is the ignorance that is all good, another the passion that is all good, and the best is the nerd-like intellectual fixation that is all good. That may sound like dumbed-down new-age Dzogchen, but if it is taken literally we can realize the inclusivity of luminous-mind Dzogchen. When we take it at face value, and truly feel stupidity, we stand confident in our flawed humanity. When passion is all good, we are free of the guilt and shame of lust and hatred, pride and jealousy, and allowing emotion to arise, unconstrained by excess, we also allow it to dissolve and vanish in spontaneous release. As for our attachment to a rational belief system, knowing that our own system is all good necessarily we admit that all belief systems are likewise included in the All-Good, and we can let go with a deep sigh of relief.

Rather than cover the earth with leather, Dudjom Rinpoche famously advised, the Dzogchen yogin wears sandals. In order to deal with all of samsara and nirvana, we need to treat the root of mind where all samsara and nirvana may be resolved. If we begin to deal with special aspects of neurosis or personality, no matter how the task is described, it becomes onerous and endless. Accepting that nothing whatsoever is excluded in the definition of the universe as "container and contents", everything has the same value. Everything that is included within the arena of inclusivity is of the nature of mind, the sameness that is the dharmakaya. Further, insofar as we admit "the root of mind", inclusivity" and "sameness" we accept responsibility for the universe, the life that inhabits it and every movement of body, speech or mind of that life. We accept responsibility for whatever has happened throughout the process of evolution. "Inclusivity" is not simply a way of positing the philosophical proposition that all experience stems from the same source, but rather a way of admitting personal responsibility for everything that we experience and, also, all the potential experience of ourselves and others.

On another level, the ramifications of inclusivity allow an all-inclusive ecumenism. In the Dzogchen view, ultimate experience of any faith – religious or secular – involves the essence of mind and whatever arises out of that essence is spontaneously perfect and that spontaneous perfection embraces the entire universe, animate and inanimate, material and spiritual, in experience of it. No matter what the color, creed or ethnicity, all are unequivocally equal. No matter what the ritual, the dogma or the god, all are united in self-aware spaciousness. The ultimate common denominator of human beings is the light of the mind. Such a view is easy for the Dzogchen adept who knows the nature of mind; but it does not serve religious believers attached to self-serving dogma, such as "The only way to do things is our way because our way is sanctioned by sacred scripture." The devotees of every religion are welcomed into the Dzogchen sangha; but Dzogchen is apostasy for fundamentalist theistic believers. Apex Dzogchen vision may include the devotees of all religions along with their beliefs and activities, but the Dzogchen view is not a formal part of all religions. We may say that all paths lead to the same final destination, but only if the Dzogchen view has been assimilated somewhere along the path. Even the techniques that are used by adepts of other faiths may be incorporated into the Dzogchen cache for appropriate and propitious prescription for sufferers in the relative world, but the Dzogchen view and meditation is unacceptable to the vast majority of religious institutions.

On the apex path no distinction is made between formal and informal contemplation and this lack of distinction allows the inclusion of everything that is experienced in every twenty-four hour period in the Dzogchen mandala. This mandala is called the "great assemblage", which can be interpreted as the entire universe assembled as an offering, or the entire universe, manifest and in potential, animate and inanimate, material and spiritual, contents and container, chalice and elixir, recognized as a plenum of experience. However it is conceived, its reality is all-inclusive. In practice this inclusivity invites every experience whatsoever into the nature of mind so that no discrimination in terms of preference or bias is allowed and no exclusion by virtue of the repression and ignorance engendered by doubt and fear.

Such a reality has no moral bias or preference and yet because it is total connectivity whatever arises is congruent with the benefit of all sentient beings. Self-serving outsiders who have heard the Dzogchen view but have not realized it experientially may indulge in self-destructive and antisocial behavior in the belief that Dzogchen sanctions it. But, in the Dzogchen view, experientially realized, nothing but compassion can eventuate.

INCLUSIVITY

"Luminous mind comprises a unity."

Just as all sunlight is considered the nature of the sun,
So all experience is the nature of luminous mind.
Identify the spaciousness of the support and location of whatever arises,
Including the entire impure, delusory universe, manifest or potential,
And everything is suffused by baseless mind and released in the now.
Reality is thus defined as the vast space of the matrix of the now,
Beyond delusion and nondelusion, beyond nominal meaning.

Even sublime self-envisioned forms and buddhafields
And the display of wholly appropriate activity in present awareness,
Are contained in the self-sprung space that is neither unity nor disunity;
Luminous mind comprises the entire universe and samsara and nirvana,
All of it noncomposite, empty clarity, like sun-dashed space,
All of it the vast, pristine, self-sprung matrix of the now.

The vast matrix of mind's nature, an unchanging skylike space,
With the creativity of luminous mind indeterminate in its display,
Governs all the lifestyles of samsara and nirvana,
The single principle of nonaction underpinning it all.
So nothing is extreme, nothing excluded or extraneous,
For nothing can stray from the reality of luminous mind.

Because everything arises as unitary, all-good spontaneity,
As an all-inclusive, unrivalled, supreme embodiment,

The greatest of the great, as all-good intrinsic spaciousness,
Like an emperor magisterially embodying the state
The whole of samsara and nirvana is passively unmoving.

Because all things are all good and not one is not good,
Undifferentiated, all things have one value in the All-Good;
Because the true and the false have one value in intrinsic spaciousness,
Everything is identical in the unmoving sameness of spontaneity.

All, without exception, arises out of the unity of intrinsic spaciousness,
Where, in nonaction, neither quest nor practice can be;
Effort and endeavor are only their own intrinsic spaciousness,
So whence could effort arise and to what could endeavor aspire?

No place to go, no vision to cultivate,
No state to attain, nothing extraneous to assimilate;
No coming nor going, the sameness of the dharmakaya,
Spontaneous perfection, lies in the spaciousness of the one sole sphere.

*

Disciples', hermits' and bodhisattvas' transmissions,
Conveying strong conviction in the absence of "I" and "mine",
Provide a shared, unelaborated, skylike vision.
The transmission of the supreme yoga, Ati, the sublime secret,
Identifies the vast space where self and other are inseparable
With the self-sprung awareness of things in the now, just as they are,
Thus including the view of the lower approaches in its supreme essence.

The three disciplines of kriya-tantra, upa-tantra and yoga-tantra,
Relating the yogin to the deity through contemplation and offering,
All aspire to the siddhi of immaculate body, speech and mind.
In the vajra-peak transmission, the sovereign secret,
Form, sound and awareness, already immaculate, comprise the deity
    of the now,
The siddhi of immaculate body, speech and mind already revealed.
The vision of the lower approaches is contained in the supreme essence.

In mahayoga, anuyoga and atiyoga, fields of yabyum deities
Constitute the universe of appearances, spiritual and material,
And since intrinsic spaciousness is inseparable
From immaculate primal awareness in the now,
Reality in its stillness is self-sprung awareness itself.
In this most sublime secret, everything is already immaculate,
And the vast uncreated matrix of the now is an actual field of bliss;
In that all-pervasive plenum without outside and inside,
No discriminating, progressive endeavor can stand,
And since everything is submerged in the now,
Liberated in the vast matrix of the dharmakaya,
Those lower visions are gathered into the secret heart of Ati.

Complete in one, complete in sum,
The matrix that contains all possible experience
Itself is contained in magnificent spontaneity,
In its intrinsic clarity, disposed in the now.

Canto Seven: Spontaneity

Introductory

Some readers may have difficulty with the usage of the word "spontaneity" in both translation and commentary. This is probably due to the intellect's demand for logical consistency in the description of experience in space-time. How can a flow or a continuum be spontaneous? Answer: it is not the flow that is spontaneous; it is every moment of awareness that is spontaneously cognizant. Awareness, then, is evinced in an endless series of discrete moments? No, because a delusive dualism of subjective awareness and objective space-time is the structure of analysis, and that duality is not a valid description of how we experience the now. In the timeless blip of awareness in the now, no distinction is made between the subjective and the objective aspect. All that we *know* in the awareness in the now is "the spontaneity". To expand that term into "spontaneous presence" is to indulge the tendency to reify the spontaneity that never crystalizes into a thing or a presence. "Pure presence", where presence is emptiness (although emptiness is inseparable from form), is an alternate way of saying "spontaneity".

In this canto, Longchenpa emphasizes the inescapable coincidence of spontaneity in the now. Spontaneity is the sole attribute (or a nonattributable verbal counter) of the now, and insofar as the now is the only thing we get, all we have ever got, and the only thing that the future will bring, it appears that spontaneity is the essential legacy of human embodiment and the nature of the great perfection. Insofar as the now is with us from conception to our last gasp spontaneity is the nature of our being, or, at least, the nature of all our experience.

Buddhists like to define spontaneity in terms of the trikaya, the three buddha bodies or the three dimensions of being, and Longchenpa follows that analytical division of ineffable, inconceivable, spontaneity – not only in this canto. The simplest way and most common way of designating the three kayas in the Dzogchen view is to define dharmakaya as emptiness, sambhogakaya as clarity and nirmanakaya as radiance. Longchenpa elaborates the dharmakaya in terms of the now. In luminous mind is the unremitting sameness of pure presence, and relaxation in the here and now reveals it. Simply leaving appearances alone reveals the clarity of the sambhogakaya. The radiance that is the nirmanakaya is noncrystallizing display, which is a pervasive matrix; it is a magical display of wishfulfilling qualities and appropriate activity. "Allowing the sediment to settle" reveals that aspect. "So given the dharmakaya as unchanging, unreferenced and all-pervasive, internal and external visions, all life forms, are the sambhogakaya and the nirmanakaya is like naturally occurring reflection."

In the moment that we recognize the vastness of our own potential, it is still our habit patterns and the tendencies that will continue to create the personality that informs our consciousness and our experience. Yet, within that experience lies the spaciousness and awareness that transcend it. If we identify with the karmic winds upon which our habit patterns ride then our activity is "instinctual". If we identify with the spaciousness of the moment, provided courtesy of our karmic propensities, then our activity will be "spontaneous". If we hang openly in the now, then lost in nondual awareness our experience will be spontaneity itself. The difference between "instinctual" and "spontaneous" (as it is used here) is the freedom in the latter from attachment to the objective field that karmic tendencies have provided us. The difference is the reifying clutch. Spontaneity itself as a denominator of nondual awareness indicates that perfectly appropriate activity is arising from the luminous nature of mind free of any personal karmic tendency.

In modern English usage the verb "to reify" generally signifies a positive move out of the amorphous night of abstraction or nonexistence into the light of day, into reality, where a sensorially perceptible object can be named and identified. The root of the nasty Latinate word "reification" is *res*, the Latin word for a "thing", so reification means "thing-ification". In Dzogchen this implies the process of turning an aspect of an experience of nonduality into "this", "that" or some other thing. The objects in the sensory fields are reified as they are objectified, in the instance of a visual perception, simultaneous with application of a label that defines a mass of nebulous color as a shape to be recognized as an entity "out there". That apparent external thing seems separate and distinct from the entity "in here" that reifies, objectifies, labels and perceives it. The mind that reifies is the intellect that grasps at objects out there, attempting to seize them and own them by clinging to them. But the intellect, the functional mind, can reify itself, and treated as an object by the dualistic consciousness that lies at the bottom of this alienating procedure, it assumes the status of a discrete entity or an island surrounded by a threatening sea. Two mountaineers scale high peaks in close proximity, but they are separated by a bottomless canyon, and recognizing in each other a similar species they can but wave to each other: the tragedy of the human predicament in samsara.

Alienated, dualistic consciousness is resolved by the simple recognition of the unitary nature of the ground of being and the illusory emanations that arise out of it. The ancient Judeo-Christian duality of man and god can be resolved in the same way – if only the priesthood sanctioned it. Regardless of the self-interest and narrowness of the priesthood, that duality is resolved in those for whom religious and linguistic convention is overtaken, because in the Dzogchen view resolution is a natural function of being, and the unitary – nondual – condition is the natural condition. The emanations of luminous mind are denominated "creativity", and as creative potential they remain identical to the luminous mind from which they cannot stray. But when creativity evolves into "display", although that display may be recognized as its primordial nature and becomes a moving picture of buddhafields, unless the adornment is experientially understood as inseparable from the luminous mind out of which it originated – if it is reified – it becomes "adornment", sensory decoration. No matter at which level dualistic perception is resolved, it is resolved in a field of sameness, where creativity, display and ornamentation are all perceived as the smoothness of a truly unitary reality.

Longchenpa takes this exposition of spontaneity as the moment to reinforce the precept of nonaction. Spontaneity is the nature of luminous mind, and insofar as spontaneity ceaselessly provides the pure presence of the now, there is no need *to do* anything. Any activity designed to facilitate or expedite the recognition of pure presence is counterproductive. Any meditative or yogic action is superfluous. Any effort is interference with an innate process. It is not so much a matter of "If it's not broken, don't fix it" but more "If you try to fix what isn't broken, you'll break it." We are already at the destination, so don't take the train. We are not going anywhere. If we have conceived of a destination, we should think again. Concerted action and effort preemptively constrain us. Intervention, no matter how benign, is disruption.

Spontaneity itself is the wish-granting agent. It provides the unity of samsara and nirvana. Don't interfere with natural spontaneity. Don't even look. If you need to pretend that you are not looking, with your hands in front of your eyes, close your eyes and avoid the temptation to glance through the chinks between your fingers. The wish-fulfilling gem is the fruition of Dzogchen.

SPONTANEITY

"Within luminous mind everything is the spontaneity of the now."

The transmission of luminous mind occurs as natural spontaneity,
It is the immediate fulfillment at the summit of Mt Meru,
The most exalted, supreme, sovereign existential modality.

When we reach the summit of a towering mountain
The lands below are visible at a glance;
From below the ambience at the peak is unknown.
Likewise, at the vajra-heart of Maha-Ati,
In the apex approach, all values are clearly apparent,
While from the lower approaches the peak is invisible:
It is the peak experience that is spontaneity.

Spontaneity is the miraculous wishfulfilling gem
That in its very nature will provide merely by the asking –
Although it is not so for dilettantish people.
The trikaya is the spontaneity in the vajra-heart,
For buddha is already accomplished in its quiescent spaciousness
Without the need of any effort or practice – therein lies its greatness.
In the lower approaches stressful discrimination is applied,
Yet nothing is accomplished for eons, except desperate neurosis.

In the now, luminous mind, the unremitting sameness of pure presence,
Left alone, just as it is, the wide-open spacious reality,
That is our dharmakaya nature, the sameness of a pristine matrix.
Present in all but recognized only by the fortunate few,
Simply by relaxing into it, its innate disposition is revealed.

As all-pervasive natural clarity, spontaneity is the sambhogakaya;
Present in all, it is the homeland seen only by a few:
Letting alone whatever manifests divulges it.

The noncrystallizing display, the nirmanakaya, is again a pervasive
    matrix;
Present everywhere, shining, clear at its inception,
It is a magical display of wishfulfilling qualities and appropriate activity,
And the matrix of immaculate intrinsic presence is like that –
Like water when the sediment has settled, natural purity revealed.

Alpha-pure experience cannot be found by conscious search,
For the buddha-high shines in a self-sprung matrix;
We need not work for it – we have it already.
Its inherent greatness is the vision of the reality-matrix:
Do not strive for what is inescapable spontaneity!

The ground of the now, gratuitous ground,
That is the ground that is the luminous heart;
Since we can never separate from our own nature
We cannot move from the pure presence of the clear light matrix!

The reason that everything is perfected by simply letting it be
Resides in the indomitable master that is fivefold pristine awareness –
Physical, energetic, mental, qualitative and active perfection, each
    fivefold –
All this is the original buddha, the spontaneity of the vast primordial
    matrix.
Do not search elsewhere – buddha is already right here!

The luminous dharmakaya of buddha, moreover,
Can be nothing other than immutable sameness;

And since it is the spontaneity of this very self-sprung space,
Don't search for it! Don't practice it! Let go of spiritual ambition!

Since the sentient beings' self-sprung awareness in the now
Remains as spontaneity in the uncontrived, unsought dharmakaya,
Without refusal or approval, enter into this spaciousness!

At the core that is unmoving, unthought, ubiquitous sameness,
The vast matrix, the ground of being, furnishes inbuilt meaning.

As immutable, ever-present, buddha in buddhafields,
We are instantly and innately empowered as buddha;
The universe is spontaneously liberated and perfect in the now,
So do not strive to make alteration – everything is already perfect,
Everything unfolding as supreme all-accomplishing spontaneity.

Canto Eight: Nonduality

Introductory

At the beginning of the twenty-first century, in the new age, the word "nondual" is a buzzword. This is a wake-up call for the Christian Church, but it also heralds new horizons in psychological theory and practice. In Dzogchen, "nondual" implies nondual perception. Nondual perception entails an inseparable unity of subjective mind, "the knower", and the objective field, or what is known. Such a unity of subject and object implies the absence of any witness in the perceptual process. No "I" controls any given situation and nor is the "I" even a passive witness to mental events. This in turn implies a thought-free mind, because thought needs to be witnessed to be conscious in the dualistic consciousness of ordinary relative mind. Nondual awareness, therefore, is something completely beyond our ability to verbalize or to express in any way whatsoever. Thus the nondual is ineffable. We could leave it there, as the most rigorous nondual schools do, but Dzogchen while assuming total nondual rigor in nonmeditation experience, in atiyoga method, allows recognition of the nondual nature of mind by means of a concept, a doorway from the dual to the nondual.

The primary verbal association with nonduality in this Dzogchen context is spontaneity, wherein spontaneity denotes (as clarified in the previous canto) a totality experience free of all causes and conditions and therefore "naturally occurring". Such an experience, of course, occurs only and uniquely in the matrix of the here and now. It occurs, then, in every moment of experience and experience itself is indeed spontaneity. Spontaneity and nonduality are the last verbal points of reference before the matrix of the now consumes us, before the final resolution.

Experientially, nonduality is said to have no point of reference. In other words the experience of nonduality cannot be said to happen, to have happened or to have a possibility of happening. Thus, nonduality, like buddha, is unknowable. If there were a point of reference, there would be a witness to it and we know "the witness" is an aspect of the subjective knower, the inner aspect of dualistic perception. If any point of reference whatsoever persists, such as a candle flame, an embodiment, a visionary panorama, spaciousness or a sense of nonduality itself, then we are still caught in the cage of dualistic perception where self and other are separate, where subjective and objective aspects are reified as distinct entities. The "unraveling" of the specific characteristics of appearances has not yet reached the place where "all distinctions are smoothed away", where a continuous state of totality obtains.

One of the antonyms of nonduality is bipolarity. If perceptual duality is the functional sensory manifestation of a loss of nondual awareness, then emotional bipolarity is its internal corollary. This emotional duality is not primary love-hate, pride-jealousy, positive-negative dualism; it is the secondary, derivative emotional polarity of hope and fear, which could be called sentiment. Our moods and thoughts can be categorized as one or the other, as either hope or fear, or somewhere on a median in between. Our belief in the concrete nature or the true existence of our hopes and fears throws us from one pole to the other. Belief in the true existence of mental phenomena is the corollary of an absence of recognition of mind's nature, an absence of contemplation. We rest in the nature of mind and although mood swings may occur, and increasingly less frequently and less excessively, we identify with the nature of the luminous mind of which they are a creative expression, and thus remain free of them.

NONDUALITY

"Luminous mind is nondual mind."

In the self-sprung awareness in the now
Where everything is singular spaciousness
Our mode of experience is essentially nondual.

A continuity of dualistic perception may arise as creative display,
But as "luminous mind" appearances and their imputation are nondual.

In the luminous, pure presence that cannot be altered or sublimated
As samsara or nirvana the universal illusion appears,
And that is to be neither abandoned nor dominated.
For the adept in whom dualistic perception is dead,
What is absent but apparent is a comic absurdity.

In its very absence, appearance shines in multifarious variety;
In its very absence, emptiness is all pervading;
In the absence of perceptual duality, we still perceive multiplicity;
In the absence of underlying substance, we still transmigrate;
In the absence of value judgment, we still distinguish pleasure and pain.

Yet looking around, people's mistakes are astounding:
Addicted to unreality as truth, they believe in a concrete reality;
Addicted to delusion as gratification, they believe in delusion;
Holding what is indeterminate as certain, they feign conviction;
Holding what is not as what is, they are foolishly credulous;
Holding what is valid as worthless, what is worthless seems validated.

With the mind preoccupied by different petty concerns,
A moment of inconsequential fixation becomes a habit
And a day, a month, a year – a lifetime – goes by unheeded.
We deceive ourselves by construing the nondual as duality.

When the adept with his pure mind looks inward,
The nameless pure presence therein, ungrounded,
Beggars description, and view and meditation are irrelevant;
Wide open, loose and spacious, in spaced-out smoothness,
There can be no sense of spiritual praxis,
No distinction between sessions and breaks in meditation,
Everything unbounded and equalized, without disruption.

Without body, object or perception as a point of reference,
Because of the smoothness of the vast expanse of the sky,
Nothing experienced within can be construed as a self.

Then looking outside at external appearances,
Everything seems evanescent, flimsy, transparent,
And disassociated, no point of reference remains.
Appearance, sound and thought, every feeling, is fresh and crisp,
And thinking, "Am I mad!" "Am I dreaming!" we burst out laughing.

Without notions of friend and foe, love and hate, close and distant
No preference for night or day, the sameness is the totality,
And samsara defined by attributes and reference points has vanished.
Without a thought of "the field of self-sprung awareness"
We have escaped the cage of belief in moral and perceptual duality.

With that realization of nondual pristine awareness
We have arrived at the self-sprung vision of the All-Good,
The place of no return, the point of consummation.

Until we realize – experientially – that field of self-sprung sameness,
We may verbally obsess with the phrase "nonduality",
And speculate confidently about what is nonreferential,
But such egregious thinking is rude and stupid.

So, in the self-sprung modality, without sublimation or alteration,
The sovereign consummate aspiration is fulfilled as nonduality;
The three realms totally liberated as nondual samsara and nirvana,
The dharmakaya citadel naturally arises within our inner nature,
And it is immaculate – "Like the sky!" we say,
Although it is actually incommensurable.

So long as we fixate on this and that as separate things,
Caught in duality, we are trapped in a cage of delusive self and other;
When, on the contrary, we make no distinction between this and that,
When all distinctions are smoothed out, points of reference gone,
Then Vajrasattva affirms that nonduality is realized.

Canto Nine: Resolution

Introductory

Western culture today is deeply riven by doubt and a sense of guilt: that is a cliché. But perhaps human beings always feel and have always felt themselves to be inadequate. The multi-billion dollar business of psychotherapy thrives upon its clients' neurotic sense of inadequacy, and the Christian Church is shored up by people's need for absolution. Perhaps the confusion attending belief in God and a failing of faith in the mystery of the crucifixion and resurrection is a corollary or a cause of this. That Longchenpa expends twice as much space on the topic of resolution as upon the previous cantos is perhaps an indication that the disease of faithlessness is endemic also in Tibet. Indeed, self-doubt and guilt (besides laughter and tears), it is said, characterize the human realm on the wheel of life.

In Dzogchen we are already in the space of buddha in buddhafields, but we do not know it. The matrix of the now is the only constant in our existence, but we do not recognize its transfiguring capacity and we do not let go of the concepts that obscure it. Resolution is what we term here recognition of the natural function of liberation. It is the spontaneous and ineluctable release of whatever arises in consciousness, release into the nature of mind out of which it arose. It is of crucial importance that we understand that this resolution is dependent upon cognition of what already exists. The resolution occurs in nonaction. Giving up our goals and our goal-oriented lifestyle and practices, rigorously eradicating the priorities on our agenda to be reached in the future and loosening the hold of deductive and inductive thinking is the corollary of relaxation into the nature of mind and its nonaction. Resolution of the gap between who we are and who we think we are is the inevitable outcome. Who we are is the vast spaciousness of awareness and clear light; who we think we are, the one who seeks liberation from the prison of samsara, is a discrete and enisled canker of consciousness composed of its history of delusory reified concepts derived from dualistic perception and then protected by fearful response as if it were a substantial entity.

This resolution is the source of the confidence that, hereafter, we can call upon to reinforce our conviction that the distinctions that arise as the creativity of the luminous mind are no different from the spacious awareness that is their intrinsic nature. Ultimately, there is no resolution, of course, because there is nothing to resolve and no one to make the resolution. This resolution, or decisive experience, is actually experience of liberation from the wheel of life, or release from the momentary, putative, object of attachment. The notion of such release can only arise within the context of confinement; if thinking of the key confirms the prison, steadfast confidence in the actuality of our freedom, wherever we may be, renders any recourse to a process of release, or a concept of release, redundant. But in the existential nexus of probability, where we have intellectual certainty and experiential equivocation, reliance upon the intuition that release is optimal in the now, that release is self-sprung and cannot be initiated or avoided, is like a lodestar, or a well of self-satisfied glee. Besides, this resolution is the resolution of every duality and that implies the resolution of bipolar prevarication, slipping between a sense of ecstatic fulfillment and tragic gloom, between certainty in our identity with buddha and the great fear of vacuity.

Resolution is built into the luminous mind that is bodhichitta. All experience, arising in luminous mind, is insubstantial, apparent yet without true existence, and as such it partakes of the nature of luminous mind. Nothing need be done to attain resolution, therefore, more than a surrender to recognition. It is misleading to identify this resolution as "sudden enlightenment", or "a decisive experience", as if it were an abrupt and incisive, life-changing experience. In the same way that a first experience of satori may indeed impinge as a sudden enlightenment experience that changes our outlook forever, resolution in Dzogchen may be an extraordinary experience, a mystical experience with light and sound effects, with dominant bliss, nonthought or clarity. But it is preeminently a nondual, zero experience. In other words it is essentially an experience without signs. It has no point of reference, so resolution cannot be identified by any sign. Likewise, resolution should not be identified with "blessing", which has as its principal attribute "bliss-waves" and which evokes a lama as its source and a devotee with faith and devotion, body and mind obeisant as its recipient. The danger, then, lies in reification of resolution. Insofar as we treat it as an experience that can be objectified, we lose it; insofar as we relax into the nonaction of the nature of mind, we secure it.

At the end of this ninth canto, which is perhaps the best verbal effusion of Dzogchen realization and the most infectious in this magnificent exposition, in the penultimate stanza, Longchenpa dwells upon the meaning of his name. For those with knowledge of Tibetan, the word *klong* in itself is less of a name than a precept, because in European languages we have no term that renders the reality that the word denotes. The "long" is the vast, spacious, nondual, spontaneous, all-inclusive arena of the now, where the now is not a fanciful metaphysical state but this actual moment of experience – right now! The "long" is the matrix. This matrix of the now provides unitary experience where pleasure – the pleasure of sensory perception – the subjective aspect is indistinguishable from the cognitive spaciousness that is its nature. The pleasure provides the author's personal name Natsok Rangdrol, "Self-releasing Multifarious Experience", and the vast matrix of the now provides his titular name, Longchenpa. Here lies an indication that we should envision Longchenpa not as an ordinary sentient being but a transcendent Guru figure equal to Kuntuzangpo. Natsok Rangdrol (or Drime Wozer, as he described himself in other colophons) is the personal finite embodiment, while Longchenpa is the impersonal body of light.

In the last stanza, Longchenpa reinforces his unprecedented very personal, individualistic foray into the intimacy of fellow being by intimating that a temporal lineage formed by himself and others, those who reside with him in the apex cockpit of the vajra-heart, carry this Dzogchen transmission. Please note that his last word in this seminal canto expresses the notion of spontaneity.

RESOLUTION

"All experience is resolved in the matrix of luminous mind."

Within the single matrix that is the vast expanse of our nature,
Skylike luminous mind is the sky-bolt,[21]
And its quintessence, its real juice,
The superlative, spacious, all-good buddha-heart
By its very nature shatters our confining shell.
In this singular supermatrix, realization and nonrealization,
Liberation and nonliberation are indivisible, sublime sameness.

The garuda bird, its wings fully developed within the egg,
The moment it hatches glides into the azure sky,
Outshining the nagas,[22] flying high above the great abyss.
So the blessed adept, realizing the vajra-heart on the apex approach,
Outshines the lesser vehicles and crosses the void of samsara.

To live in the supreme sameness that is total liberation,
Inimical to those on the path of goal-oriented endeavor,
Validates the immutable sameness of the supreme approach.

Everything is blissful in this skylike dharmakaya matrix;
In this dharmakaya matrix, nothing remains unliberated;
Reality divulges itself as the sublime forms of the vajra-heart,
While the karmically generated body is the heart's perfect creativity.
When the conditioned body is abandoned in the bardo of life
Everything is pure presence alone, in no way divisible;
With the mastery of the victors on the level of spontaneity
Emanation emerges without any restriction
And every situation is embraced without impediment.
"To ride the winds", effortlessly, defines the adept's career,
And although, of course, it is inimical in the lower approaches.
Ati accepts it as the crux of fruition,

Birth occurs as unborn magical emanation,
While the fickle intellect fixates on causal relations:
Ati reveals unconditional noncausality,

And what is inadmissible in the lower approaches
Here becomes the crux.

Buddha and sentient beings, the vision and the actuality, inseparable,
It is the deluded intellect that holds samsara and nirvana apart:
Ati reveals nonduality,
And what is discordant in the lower approaches
Here becomes the crux.

Realization and nonrealization equally released,
To believe in release through realization denies their equality:
Ati reveals unitary sameness
And what is unacceptable in the lower approaches
Here becomes the crux.

Only an idiot relies upon a specific method of attainment
For ineffable – nonspecific – realization:
Ati reveals ultimacy to be indivisible
And what is inimical to the lower approaches
Here becomes the crux.

All pervasive in the now, Dzogchen is measureless,
But it is only the idiot who calls it nebulous:
Ati shows unbounded immediacy
And what is disagreeable in the lower approaches
Here becomes the crux.

In the one sole sphere the linear, causal, process is reversed,
And skylike sameness unravels goal-related hope and fear.
It is vast, it is magnificent – skylike buddha-mind!
Without goal-fixation – the matrix of the one sole sphere!
Liberation in the now – whether or not we are realized!
Happy the yogin on the skylike path of nonaction!

This objectless pure presence of buddha in the now
Supersedes the delusory ground and the roaming in samsara –
No one can be deluded because no place of delusion exists.
Here everything is intrinsic spaciousness in a single matrix of clarity;

Free of linear time, it is skylike open spaciousness,
The spontaneity of alpha-pure samsara disposed in the now.

There can be no "attaining liberation" or "entering nirvana",
For samsara and nirvana are unknown in the immutable supermatrix
And moral preference, hope and fear, are unimaginable
In the primordially luminous ground, in that vast matrix.
All things are mere label, in reality unutterable,
So neither liberation nor delusion can exist,
And samsara and nirvana are already resolved.
Make no effort! Do not try to change things!

Pure presence has no breadth or depth, no high or low,
And this boundless indeterminacy precludes any point of reference;
Pure presence has no agenda, nothing to do and nowhere to go,
And the absence of linear time and antidote precludes goal-fixation.
Any contrived point of reference results in captivity,
So setting no goals whatsoever, relax into the totality!

*

Whether or not our experience is released in the now,
Whether or not our way of being is pure in its nature,
Whether or not the nature of mind is discursively elaborated,
Whether or not we bathe in the genuine authentic disposition,
It is all the same.

Whether or not we see samsara and nirvana as a duality,
Whether or not all thought and expression is transcended,
Whether or not delusive logical thinking has been eradicated,
Whether or not the existential view has been actualized,
It is immaterial.

Whether or not we live in contemplation of reality,
Whether or not we live without discrimination,
Whether or not we live natural perfection as fruition,
Whether or not we have traversed the levels and paths,
It is all beside the point.

Whether or not we are free of all obscuration,
Whether or not creative and fulfillment stages have completed our
    reality,
Whether or not release has been attained as fruition,
Whether or not we wander in samsara's six mythic realms,
It makes no difference.

Whether or not the nature of our being is spontaneity,
Whether or not dualistic assertion and negation bind us,
Whether or not we have arrived at the ultimate vision of reality,
Whether or not we follow in the footsteps of our master –
It does not matter.

No matter what occurs, even if the sky and the earth change places,
We are wide open, hanging loosely, authentic in groundlessness;
Without reference, disassociated, evanescent, randomized,[23]
Without either hope or fear we are uninhibited, divinely mad;
View and meditation identical, the intellect's fixations collapse,
And we are free of wishful thinking and goal-orientation
And nothing to strive for or to practice remains.

Whatever happens let it happen; whatever manifests let it shine,
Whatever arises let it dawn and whatever occurs just let it be;
And, moreover, whatever is anything let it be nothing at all.

*

Our behavior become unpredictably varied,
We are thrust immediately into pure presence
Where computation of truth and untruth has no ground;
Without reference, in boundless transparence, beyond the trap of
    philosophy,
Eating, moving, sleeping, sitting, day and night, a smooth continuum,
We live in the sameness of the reality of our own nature.

With no gods to worship, no spirits to exorcise,
No culture of meditation, in an unpretentious free and easy state,
Here is an unaffected lord without pride in his sense of totality,

And wide open, hanging loosely, in spontaneity and oneness,
Without need to act, secure in the now, stress-free, he is happy.

The view is without ground and meditation is not a "state",
So, there is no discipline to pursue and no goal to attain;
No preference anywhere, all distinctions smoothed away,
Without need of stress or strain, in zero dimension, we are content.

In the absence of ambition, all disciplined practice ends,
And with nothing to lose, we let go of remedial strictures;
Since neither something, nor everything, nor nothing exists,
Whatever appears, whatever occurs, is already released;
Since no release, by nature, in the now, or by itself is possible,
The unreferenced totality has gone beyond resolution.

So vast the matrix, so vast, a supermatrix, the spaciousness of space,
In this all-embracing supermatrix,[24] an all-saturating matrix of clarity,
Bliss and matrix swept into one unitary, nondual matrix,
All things whatsoever are self-released,[25] and reality is consummate.
Unchangeable spontaneity is what I most desire for us all.

Moreover, all of us, all those who follow my example,
Merging the all-embracing now with the supermatrix,[26]
We have mastery on the level of the All-Good!

Canto Ten: Vision

Introductory

Some will consider this tenth canto on vision to be the heart of Longchenpa's treatise. Certainly, if any of the thirteen cantos could be considered a statement of method, it is this one. It may be argued that no method is to be pursued in the vajra-heart, except recognition of what is already present. Atiyoga, surely, is a method of simply pointing out ineluctable reality, a conceptual introduction to what is nonconceptual and beyond the intellect to comprehend. That is precisely what this *Treasury of the Dharmadhatu* does – it "points out" and it "introduces". But in this canto we are urged to retain the vision of mind's nature, and since retention implies extension in time, that surely is an ongoing activity, a practice. In the last verse of the canto, in which Longchenpa moderates his style to introduce an avuncular tone to give personal advice to his students, he confirms that nothing is to be done in atiyoga other than to keep the vision – "Keep the faith!" He does not qualify that statement with the sophistic assertion that maintaining the vision is nothing but relaxing into the space of nonaction – but he might have done!

In the same verse at the end of the canto, Longchenpa stresses that this guru-vision of reality is the outcome of the resolution of cause and effect, of causality, and the affectivity of secondary conditions. That assertion may tempt some people to exert themselves in undermining the space-time assumptions that inform our thinking, belief systems and language. Our linguistic structure itself, surely, describes a dualistic delusion in which the creativity of luminous mind has become crystallized as the adornment that we know as the animate and inanimate universe (although this may not be true of the structure of all languages). How can we recognize the creativity of mind as its own luminous essence if we have not excised the kind of thinking that links the past with the present and the present with the future, and in the present envisages the universe in terms of the four cardinal and the eight intermediate directions, top and bottom existing in a temporal continuum? Surely, reality is a nondual spaciousness where center and circumference are identical. The answer to this lies in the proposition Longchenpa articulated in the previous canto, that the resolution of every dualism occurs naturally and spontaneously because it is the natural function of mind. This assertion is repeated in the eleventh canto treating release. In the resolution of duality the vision is naturally and spontaneously displayed. Thus, again, although Longchenpa employs the word "method" to describe the resolution into guru-vision, is this notion appropriate?

In the penultimate line of the final stanza of this tenth canto, a stanza containing what are known as core secret precepts, Longchenpa evokes the notion of the "excluded middle". Aristotle, a Greek, first formulated the law of excluded middle. He maintained therein that in response to any proposition it is necessary to either affirm or deny, that irrefutable logic disallowed any "middle" response that neither affirmed nor denied. Thus, for example, the proposition that "life is suffering" must receive a veritable yea or nay, and any response such as Nagarjuna's fourfold negation – not yea, not nay, neither both yea and nay, nor neither yea nor nay – was illogical and unacceptable. Nagarjuna's fourfold negation, of course, presents the logical case for the excluded middle. Here "spaciousness" may be existentially experienced. So the excluded middle is what in Dzogchen we may term the ineffable reality of the here and now, in its emptiness, clarity and compassion.

This guru-vision is direct perception of the here and now and is therefore a nondual vision and cannot be described in dualistic terms. It is crucial that we do not consider that this vision is a preview of what we intend to attain in the future when we have "accumulated the merit", "purified our karma", "done the necessary preliminaries" and so on. The vision is valid only in the here and now and only for the timeless moment of its experience.

In order to fulfill this guru-vision, the view and the meditation must remain integrated. It may appear at first that the view is a series of highly abstract intellectual statements describing a hypothetical reality. But soon those statements become immediately actualized precepts

– the precepts are actualized as nonmeditation. The view provides doorways into experiential Dzogchen, and that is nonmeditation. The great temptation is to turn nonmeditation into a discipline on a progressive path, in which case view and meditation remain asunder. Confidence derived from initiatory experience is imperative at this moment and the support of a rigzin-lama is crucial. If we can retain confidence in the view, then we rest in meditation, and view and meditation are nonmeditation. If we lose confidence in the view then we are stuck with shamata and vipasyana meditations on the gradual path of Tibetan cultural learning.

We may find it surprising, then, that Longchenpa's auto-commentary on this the tenth canto, the most extensive and detailed of all, elaborates the precepts that are crucial in atiyoga – in trekcho and togal. We know that these precepts are crucial to discovering the nonmeditation that is the key to Maha-Ati, but still Longchenpa's auto-commentary leaves a taste of the progressive method. The first set of precepts is called the four modes of freely resting; the second is called the three aspects of contemplation; and the third is called the twenty-two topics. What are these twenty-nine topics that Longchenpa lists in his commentary? They may be considered as twenty-nine conceptual keys to nonconceptual experience. In a certain way, they are paradoxes that in their resolution produce a transcendent response. Perhaps, sometimes, that response could be called nondual and in that they are very similar to the Rinzai-zen koans. But these Dzogchen precepts are to be resolved in simply sitting, by a natural relaxation into the nature of mind, and not by any arduous process of sadhana. The assumption, here, is that the concept itself, implicit in the precept, is congruent with the experience and that the nature of the experience is the underlying, all-pervasive experience of the spaciousness that is present in the natural state of being. If, indeed, this vision of Dzogchen describes the intrinsic reality of all our lives then the concept of it becomes a doorway into its realization.

The freely resting precepts demonstrate a paradigm of atiyoga method. If we take "mountain" as an example, we are not exhorted to do anything with this mountain, not to visualize it, outside or inside, not to identify our minds with it, not to cultivate its qualities of immobility, solidity, immutability and so on, nor even to enumerate its qualities. Recognition is the keyword and that is not to be considered "an action" under this atiyoga rubric. Rather, it is "nonaction". Then consider another of the freely resting precepts, "ocean", a concept representing the eternal sea. Simply by allowing the notion "ocean" to arise in the mind, we dwell in the ocean and are engulfed by the ocean, and the symbolic value of the ocean evokes its clarity, unity, stillness and vastness. In recognition we know the spaciousness of luminous mind. Again, no action is to be performed here, no contrivance or fabrication, but rather we are recognizing the nature of mind that has existed prior to our perception and what is called the natural state of being.

Further, "ocean" as a symbol may also evoke a cresting wave, like Hokusai's *Great Wave*, where the foam of the ocean appears to be have strayed from the ocean itself, the separation belied by the certain knowledge that it will fall back into the ocean in the next moment. Just as that Japanese painting first evokes samsara in all its threatening alienation, and then in the next instant provides the comforting, calming knowledge that the boat and its occupants will survive, so knowing oneself as the ocean may first evoke samsara and then nirvana within it and bring that gratuitous consummation in nonduality.

The stanza in the root text, the third stanza, to which this freely resting example is attached, stresses the ocean's stillness and pellucidity. That indicates a state of mind where no alternation between the mental projection of an image or object and that image's collapse can be. Externally that identity occurs in the process of rising and falling of sensory imagery and internally in the process of elaboration of perception into streams of thought and its dissolution. Or are these processes better described as timeless "pulsations" of mind? The commentary focuses upon the experience of a still ocean with the reflections of the planets and stars shining within it, giving it much the same significance as the reflection of the moon in water, which is one of the eight classical analogies of reality.

After this analysis of the modes of freely resting, it must be stressed that no "state" exists to be achieved. Thinking that Dzogchen is a state to be realized, immediately reifies Dzogchen and emphasizes the duality that is to be resolved. So any thought that pure presence is a state like elation or depression, or certainty or doubt, is to be experientially deconstructed at the moment of its arising just like every discursive thought – any belief – that arises. If pure presence were a definable state, there would be a cause and conditions that effected that state, and there would be an effect that was caused subsequently by that state. If pure presence was caused by certain conditions then the formalization of those conditions as technique would allow us to practice it, in a process, on a path that led to the destination, the goal, which would be a fixed state. That state would appear to "truly exist" in space-time; but since it would be a product of causality it would be composite and therefore impermanent and a part of conditioned existence, which is another name for samsara. In the samsaric realm where zealous ambition is required to attain any worthwhile goal, shades of jealousy and rivalry inevitably transpire, even in the most purified minds, because goal-orientation accompanied by ambition is generally attended by contention. Constant concern with the stage of the path and the degree of attainment would upset the mind, and, finally, "the state" cannot be attained due to concern whether or not it had been attained. Longchenpa is adamant that there is no state of mind to be achieved. To allow the concept of "the state" on the grounds that it is the state of nondual cognition in contradistinction to the dualistic state of perception is to overindulge the intellect. It is as if the intellect were just waiting for the pronouncement of "a state" in order to reify it and then to grasp it, to cling to it, to defend and justify itself through it. The thought and concept, then, either precede or supersede the actual experience. If the concept precedes it, then it is the penetration of the thought by primal awareness from within that allows the experience; if the concept was subsequent to the experience then dualistic perception has already muddied the waters.

Just by thinking, "This is it!" "This is the state!" then we have lost it, because the state cannot be objectified and reduced to a mere label. If we add insult to injury and to our *eureka* pronouncement, add an intention to remain in that state, thinking, "How can I remain in this state?" and we manage to fixate the state and sustain it, then what is stabilized is a trance state. As often quoted, a trance state is the meditation of the gods, or perhaps a samadhi of the Hindu rishis, or a fixation of the Buddhist meditator who has gone astray. The natural state of authentic being, which is the situation when we rest doing nothing – abandoning nothing nor adopting nothing – has no witness and therefore cannot be established or recollected. The self-sprung awareness that is the reality of that moment has no attributes or characteristics. So how can it be called "a state"? And who is there to verify the nature of that state? Who is the witness? Is it possible that someone on the outside can actually verify another person's state of mind? It may be possible to confirm the probability of someone else's insistent report of an ineffable state, but such a report can describe only its passing, like the tail of a comet that provides evidence of the invisible body that preceded it. The Dzogchen adept can never provide evidence of his nondual awareness; for that reason alone he may be anonymous.

It must be stressed and reiterated that, in the vision, there can never be any distraction, obstacle or error. What we call a distraction from a particular object of focus is defined by reference to a predetermined fixation, while in the vision the distraction has already become the subject of nonmeditation. Likewise, although in Vajrayana obstacles and obscurations may be taken as the path, in this Dzogchen vision no limiting notions such as "obstacles" and "obscurations" can arise. There are no goals and no preconceived causal functions, so whatever occurs, perfect as it is, is the vast spaciousness of the now. There can be no error in reality. Everything that arises in the vision of reality is perceived immediately as perfect in itself, and known as a field of sameness wherein nothing has any greater virtue than anything else. Furthermore, there can be no error because there is no one to define right and wrong and no one to set a bias that prefers one thing to another. There is no error because error in itself is the nature of mind, a vast matrix of spaciousness. There is no error because relative and absolute truth are one reality; every moment of our consciousness in the here and now demonstrates that. Only when the intellect in its mode of dualistic perception separates absolute from relative can the notion of an ideal state of consciousness distinct from the present moment arise. And there is the crux of the delusion of samsara: the thought that something achievable exists, a goal exists to be won – out there or in here – a state superior to what we have in the now, necessarily exacerbates the pain and sadness that originally motivated such a thought. The dissatisfaction that motivates desire for improvement carries with it an endless cycle of dissatisfaction. Caught in that eternal loop, we suffer the cyclic round of samsara, rebirth and delusion. At the inception of every thought, before it is apprehended, is the clarity and emptiness of the dharmakaya, the spaciousness of mind's nature, and therein no error or mistake can be made.

Finally, in this tenth chapter treating vision, here is a digression upon the notion of reincarnation. For the Dzogchen adept, in the instantaneous process of disillusionment that is every timeless slice of the here and now, the notion of rebirth, like all beliefs, must be existentially deconstructed. Like each sensory perception, inner or outer, like every thought as it arises, the notion of reincarnation is to be unraveled and spread out, so that it is understood as its reality-constituent – spaciousness. As such, we know it as sameness, the same spaciousness as all thought and, indeed, all perception. In that knowing, we relieve ourselves of attachment to particular thought-forms and attain the faculty to utilize all beliefs according to people's needs. It may offend some Buddhists, but our attachment to all particular thought-forms is to be released, and that includes the notion of rebirth.

The notion of rebirth is apparently as deeply entrenched in the Indian sub-continent as the concept of heaven and hell must have been in medieval Europe. In the sixth century B.C, at the time of Sakyamuni Buddha, transmigration after death was almost certainly universally accepted. We may assume that because the notion of rebirth was a basic unquestioned assumption about existence to doubt it was to throw oneself into social and religious disrepute. Rather than argue the case in his popular preaching, Sakyamuni preferred not to address the issue, and for that reason it is not treated in the exoteric sermons that were later to be enshrined in the canonical sutras. "If we follow the eightfold path in this lifetime, whatever happens after death will take care of itself in the best possible way", was his teaching. If we replace "follow the eightfold path" with "relax into the nature of mind" this is very much the attitude in Dzogchen. Rebirth is just another obdurate belief, like belief in the flat earth; like the belief in a substantial, weighty soul; like belief in the superiority of the white race; like belief that the sun encircles the earth; like belief in the big bang at the beginning of time; like belief in the internal combustion engine; and like belief in contemporary aerodynamics. Just as it is extremely injudicious, however, to assert absolutely the absence of causality when in the next moment samsara may clamp down and ignorance of the law of cause and effect place us in a perilous pass, the lower-realm abyss yawning open beneath us, or perhaps when in a flash of insight we see that samsara is indisputably the creativity of luminous mind, so it is foolish to deny adamantly the possibility of rebirth. The continuity of space-time in this life, after all, does appear to be broken occasionally by a metaphysical death and subsequent rebirth, as the Dzogchen instruction in the bardos – the intermediate states – implies. We can only say that in the light of the nondual matrix of the here and now there can be no rebirth, although in the unpredictable and variable emanations of space-time anything and everything is possible.

VISION

"Guru-vision is identical to true reality."

Luminous mind with its alpha-pure nature,
The invariable reality that has nothing to expunge or espouse,
A skylike matrix, a reality that cannot be sought and found,
Shines as stellar light simply as we rest in its nature.

The sensory fields do not crystalize here, mind is not reified,
And unmoving from essential spontaneity,
We arrive at the guru-vision of the all-good vast expanse.

*

Crystal clear space, free of alternation and pulsation,
Like a still, unsullied, translucent ocean,
In the simple clear reality of self-sprung awareness in the now,
We rest free of fluctuating hope and fear.

In a preverbal space where there are no habitual compulsions,
Naturally disposed, unfeigned, uncontrived and unalloyed,
Yes, absorbed by the matrix into the reality that has no attribute,
Neither meditation nor anything to meditate upon can be.
Bipolarity set free becomes the self-sprung reality-vision.

All basic thought patterns are the creativity of pure presence,
So, renounced they may be, but they cannot be eliminated;
In their reality, no differentiation or exclusion, no distinction, can exist,
So, may be present, but they cannot be definitively established;
And their true reality is known simply as their spaciousness.

Without rejecting samsara, we see it as self-sprung awareness in the now,
Envisioned through pure authenticity as the creativity of the
   supermatrix.

In the now, sensory appearances and mind fall together as reality,
Where still contemplation occurs in an uninterrupted flow.
This is the vajra-peak, the supreme all-good buddha-mind,
The most sublime spacious event, as high as the sky.
Without differentiation or exclusion, the supreme meditation
Invests the now, the marvelous lord that is spontaneity.

*

In the now, empowering clear light is a continuum,
A spontaneity wherein nothing is expunged or espoused –
This is the supreme vision of samsara and nirvana as spaciousness.
This skylike supermatrix itself, unmoving and ineffable,
In the now, is the natural disposition of all beings.

Seeing appearances as other than oneself is mental delusion;
Belief in meditation and endeavor is mental delusion.
The true reality of delusion is a field of sameness, a state of rest,
But in that matrix that is unmoving and alpha-pure,
There can be no action or endeavor, no resting nor nonresting.

Looking at the reality that is unchanging spontaneity
With its intrinsic presence that is free of intellectual interference,
Looking again and again, we see nothing –
Nonseeing is the empowering view of pure presence.

In the undiscriminating pure presence that cannot be cultivated,
Pursuing meditation, we see nothing exists to meditate upon –
Nonmeditation is the empowering meditation of pure presence.

In the nondual way of being that is free of discrimination,
In disciplined conduct, we see nothing exists to practice –
Nondiscipline is the empowering conduct of pure presence.

Secure in the now, in the spontaneity free of hope and fear,
In repetitive accomplishment, we see no accomplishment –
Nonaccomplishment is the empowering accomplishment of pure
    presence.

*

In sameness objects are not conceptualized,
Nor is mind reified, so fluctuating hope and fear subside;
Living in the space where object and mind are identical
Reality never moves out of the matrix,
Nothing is objectified in the field of attributes,
And so, thereby, we are empowered.
In the now, through its nondual empowering awareness,
The great perfection, inseparable samsara and nirvana,
Without any giving or taking is an all-pervasive smoothness.

Matter and spirit are the same in intrinsic spaciousness,
And buddha and sentient beings are the same in intrinsic spaciousness,
And absolute and relative are the same in intrinsic spaciousness,
And sin and virtue are the same in intrinsic spaciousness,
And the ten directions[27] are all the same in intrinsic spaciousness.
Consequently, everything arising as self-sprung display,
At its inception, all the same, nothing ever better or worse,
What is the use of positive or negative antidotes?
In their abiding, all things are the same, nothing ever better or worse,
So let whatever arises in the mind subside into itself right now!
In their release, all things are the same, nothing ever better or worse,
So in the aftermath, why make any judgment?

Everything arising as luminous mind in the ground of being,
Arising as creativity or display, it is all indeterminate:
Arising equally undetermined in the original matrix of the now,
Though it may seem to arise unambiguously,
Everything arises as the sameness of intrinsic spaciousness;
Again, everything existing the same at rest in reality,
Though dissimilarity may appear to exist
Everything abides in the sameness of intrinsic spaciousness;
And again, released, self-sprung in the matrix of primal awareness,

Even though it may not appear to be released,
It is actually released in the total sameness of spaciousness.

In self-sprung presence, everything the same in the now,
Arising or nonarising
Everything is always absent in intrinsic spaciousness;
Abiding or nonabiding
Everything is always absent in intrinsic spaciousness;
Released or unreleased
Everything is always absent in intrinsic spaciousness.

In the pure presence of immutable sameness,
At inception, spontaneously arising,
Everything is known in its intrinsic state;
As it abides, spontaneously abiding,
Everything is known in its intrinsic state;
And at dissolution, spontaneously dissolving,
Everything is known in its intrinsic state.

In pure presence unchanging and unelaborated,
Everything arising arises in the now,
Everything abiding abides in the now,
Everything dissolving is released in the now,
And its nature is like the sky.

*

Coincident arising, abiding and release is an uninterrupted flow –
No break in the arising and dissolving is possible;
In an unbroken stream cause and effect are inseparable,
And because causality is inoperable, the abyss of samsara is crossed,
And if the abyss is traversed, downfall is avoided.

The matrix of Samantabhadra is the unvarying now;
The matrix of Vajrasattva is incapable of alteration or sublimation;
Simple recognition of the nature of being is labeled "buddha".

With that realization, nothing to adopt or abandon,
Everything is smoothed into its unique reality –

On the Isle of Gold all things must be gold.
Where there are no parameters, no limitations,
Deviation is impossible and veils are transparent;
So in luminous mind, no downfall possible,
The three dimensions are spontaneously, effortlessly, complete
And the phrase "unimaginable and inexpressible" a mere figure of speech.

Sensory appearances undone, pure presence self-sprung shines out,
And unveiled, without inside or outside, appearances are transparent –
In genuine, natural disposition, everything shines in supreme reality.
Relaxing our bodymind in satisfaction,
Hanging loose, like someone who has nothing to lose,
Neither tense nor slack, the bodymind rests comfortably.

*

No matter how we feel, we abide in the nature of mind;
No matter how we live, we stay in the nature of mind;
No matter how we move, we move in the nature of mind.
In luminous spaciousness, coming and going are impossible –
No movement in the victors' dimension!

Whatever we say reverberates as mind's nature;
Whatever is expressed is articulated as mind's nature:
In luminous mind no verbal expression manifests,
For the speech of the victors is ineffable.

Whatever ideas emerge are thought as the nature of mind;
Whatever concepts emerge are conceived as the nature of mind:
In luminous mind ideas and concepts never truly exist
For the mind of the victors is a thoughtless mind.

Absence occurring as anything at all is the nirmanakaya;
Enjoyment in the nature of mind is the sambhogakaya;
The absence of any substantial ground therein is the dharmakaya:
The three dimensions as fruition comprise the spontaneity-matrix.

In the spacious supermatrix of luminous mind
No discursive thought arises;

If the ordinary mind is untrammelled by signs of perception,
That is the vision of holistic buddha.

Luminosity, in essence like the spacious vault of the sky,
Without thought or concept, is the supreme meditation;
Luminosity, in essence like the spacious vault of the sky,
Without thought or concept, is the supreme meditation,

Nothing but our own nature unmoving and uncontrived,
Without mentation, nothing at all generated in the mind,
That is reality, naturally disposed, nothing changing in time,
The supreme meditation, where the movement of thought ceases.

Whatever rests in that intrinsic nature is sacred, fearless mind;
It is holistic buddha, free of all attributes;
It is unmoving spaciousness that equalizes all reifying concepts;
It is the victors' vision-matrix, the supreme expanse of our being.
Abandoning the chains of fabricated bodymind,
In unfeigned relaxation, regardless of any stirring thought-forms,
When we abide in the ground of being and stay in that reality,
Everything is the vast all-good vision-matrix.

*

Free of the stress of compulsive give and take,
We are uninhibited, naturally disposed in our very being;
The matrix without parameters is a still all-pervasive smoothness,
And all thought-forms subsiding by themselves into themselves,
That is Vajrasattva's skylike vision.

If we are undistracted from the authentic matrix of luminous mind,
Though we engage with the mental field, that is also reality;
But if that reality is adulterated by any compulsiveness,
Although the matrix is thoughtfree and spacious like the sky,
We are caught in a cage of reified concepts.
We may meditate continuously in that way – but it is mere trance,
And trance, said Sakyamuni, is similar to the meditation of the gods.
So it is crucial that mind is undistracted and without motivation,
Remaining in its natural disposition, transcending goal-orientation.

Since self-sprung awareness in the now is zero-dimensional,
No "thing" or "goal" or "ideal" is ever indicated therein,
For all mental elaboration has naturally collapsed.
Intellectual stratagems and rational agendas have been abandoned
And we familiarize ourselves with the sublime groundless expanse.

The one holistic reality is self-sprung awareness in the now;
The one holistic view is free of discursive opinions;
The one holistic meditation neither lacks nor wants nothing;
The one holistic conduct comprises nondual giving and taking;
The one holistic fruition detests moral preference:
That is the self-sprung guru-vision of spontaneity.

The universe, material and spiritual, samsara and nirvana –
All experience whatsoever is reality from the first;
Since it cannot stray from self-sprung awareness itself,
All experience is disposed as the ground of being:
That is guru-vision.

*

Regarding reality appearing as a multifarious field,
Without worrying about any preceptual disposition,
Simply rest in naturally disposed, nonpulsating mind,
And we stay naturally in the reality that is the matrix of sameness.

Regarding the forms of sensory appearance in a field of duality,
By neither focusing the senses nor letting the gaze wander,
Free of a sense of "self" or an idea of "other",
We allow natural clarity to shine in vast smoothed-out openness.

In the vision of all-identical, self-sprung awareness in the now,
Where free of pulsation, mind is expanded and heightened,
Experiencing integral space free of outside, inside and in between,
Blissful, clear contemplation, free of discursive elaboration, arises.

*

Regarding the vision of reality unmoving in the quiescent ground,
No outside, no inside, exists, no elaboration of perceptual duality,

And since there is no mind that fixates "objects" as other,
Nothing exists to get hold of and no attachment to perception,
And nowhere in samsara to take rebirth – there is only the sky!

When the mind is not conceived as "oneself" within,
There is nothing to grasp and nothing to become attached,
And all habitual assumptions about conditioned existence subside,
And the "person" to be reborn in samsara vanishes.
At this point, where outer and inner are both like the sky,
Delusive experience cannot be conceived or imagined,
And we have arrived at the dharmakaya vision.
Touching final resolution, coming and going now barred,
We reach the supreme citadel of the dharmakaya,
The pure fields of the All-Good, the all-saturating matrix.

If pure presence of the now does not stray from the ground of being,
Familiarization with it precludes strengthened conditioned existence
And the karma and habit that perpetuate rebirth run dry;
Causality resolved, we say that samsara and nirvana are identical,
And being in neither conditioned existence nor peaceful cessation
We have arrived at the luminous-heart core,
That is definitely not a state of one-pointed calm abiding[28] –
It is the vision of natural great perfection.

When we vacillate, losing the essential grounded space,
The intellectual mind at work becomes samsara itself,
Involving causal concatenation that precludes resolution,
And, inevitably, we fall lower and lower.
The supreme secret, the great perfection, on the other hand,
Never strays from intrinsic spaciousness
And the forms of its creativity naturally dissolve into their source:
This vision is the vision of immutable sameness.

In this vision, goal-directed endeavor is impossible,
So, the view, for example, cannot be cultivated;
Yet, out of this space where center and circumference are unified
Creativity projects its display into another dimension,
Where it appears as the multifarious variety of the universe:
Never say categorically that cause and effect do not exist!

The complexity that arises from interdependence is incalculable;
The states of samsaric delusion and nirvanic joy are incalculable:
A mass of causes and conditions constitutes a sublime synchronicity.

When we identify our authentic nature, nothing can be said about it;
Likewise, taking authenticity as the path, wholly committed,
Knowing it only in moments of unimaged, nonconceptual vision,
Consumed by it, we are completely, transparently, naked.

*

In this supermatrix, afflictive emotion, karma and habit
Create apparitional games of magical illusion.
To be free of that, please, we resolve causality.
Our method is supreme:
Never, never stray from the vision of reality,
And cherish the excluded middle!²⁹
That is the crux of my heartfelt advice.

Canto Eleven: Purity

Introductory

Purity is a close synonym of emptiness. Purity is the pellucid cleanliness of a moving mountain stream. Purity is the nature of the sky and the nature of the spaciousness of all human experience. So what is a "pure" situation? A "pure" event? Certainly it is nothing to do with morality. Any and every experience is rendered pure, says Longchenpa, by the intrinsic purity of cognition. He is referring to the cognition that is implied in pure presence. Purity lies in both the spaciousness of the objective aspect of consciousness and the spaciousness of its internal, subjective aspect; but these two aspects are one in the experiential knowing of the now. Purity is thus another word for luminous mind.

To image this pure unitary experience of the now, we can turn to togal, or rather to the reality of the unity of trekcho and togal. Here the notion of "a smoothed-out" field of illusory color and shape, a field in which all distinctions have been removed yet retaining a slight hint that something might still be there, serves to invoke the togal vision. That smoothed-out field is the sameness of all experience. In the same way, consider a process of constant – momentary – unraveling of the objective aspect of sensory perception so that an illusion of a constant plenum of purity appears, although some vestiges of what has been unraveled remain. Certainly, that plenum of purity is not a spacious vacuum, and yet nothing substantial – not even a Higgs' boson – exists there. What, indeed, remains when the complexities of intellectually-informed perception unravel themselves, whether that perception is a seemingly external objective field of sub-nuclear particles, or an internal field of mental consciousness? Perhaps the vestiges of such perceptions could be best described as a "pixelated" field. Just as the pixels of an LCD screen are the invisible (at a distance) basis of a multicolored visual, so the spaciousness of appearances is revealed to the senses. The unraveling of seemingly concrete entities is the trekcho part, while the perception of the pixelation is the togal part, and of course these two parts are one.

This "pixelated field" nicely synthesizes trekcho and togal vision. It describes the totality-vision of pure presence that is intrinsic spaciousness but gives equal ontological status to the emptiness aspect and its brilliance. This brilliance is what is sometimes perceived, and then described, in terms of *thig-les* and it is in that concept where the notion of pixels has its source. In the same way that pixels comprise a photograph or a computer screen, so in an organic three-dimensional construct they comprise every visual field. It is that field that is indicated in togal as the visible pure presence. It is the same field that is indicated in trekcho as nondual spaciousness. Thus the phrase "spaced out in pixelation" may describe the mode of Vajrasattva!

Nonaction is a primal Dzogchen notion that Longchenpa desisted from enshrining in a canto of its own, but nevertheless gave it space in all cantos. This canto may appear to treat precepts on meditation, but Longchenpa in his auto-commentary considers it to be instruction on conduct. He gives it the title "Resting in Uncontrived Conduct". Uncontrived conduct is a synonym of nonaction. Nonaction subsumes all conduct, all activity, all behavior. Nonaction includes all and any activity whatsoever. But then nonaction is like the illusion of a static hub lying within the revolving wheel of a moving vehicle. The precepts articulated in this canto, although they may appear to be describing particular mental activity, are actually like that static wheel-hub of the moving vehicle – the functions described are all attributes of the natural state of mind, which is achieved only by doing nothing. "Recognition" is not to be considered an action and its qualities cannot be reified. It is all pure presence.

In this eleventh canto, Longchenpa mentions the natural tendency to secrecy. Secrecy is the automatic function of pure presence because of an innate understanding that any commentary upon the heart teaching is inevitably interpretive – surely any intellectual processing of experience of the here and now is interpretive and therefore derogatory – and the feeling-tone of an exaggerated appreciation of mind's nature is at variance with the guru-vision. Buddha realization and its simultaneous articulation fall outside the stricture against secrecy. The tendency of the adept to share experience of mind's nature verbally with those who have not been so lucky dissolves at its inception in the purity of pure presence.

PURITY

"All situations are pure like the sky."

Within the unitary luminous mind, everything the same as the sky,
Dualistic perception deludes us with causal, conditioned existence;
Appreciating those baseless delusory appearances as magical illusion
Through direct perception, calculation preempted, no trace remains.

When anger, dismay, envy, trouble or irritation,
Anxiety, depression or mental pain,
Fear of death and rebirth, and so on,
Accompanies negative reaction to unwelcome events,
Recognize it at its inception as a display of creative power.
Do not reject it or indulge it, do not try to purify or alter it,
But, rather, without applying view or meditation,
In the naturally disposed smoothed-out totality,
Free of pulsating thought and image, rest without self-consciousness.
The self-dissolving, traceless, sky-matrix of expansive mind
Then dawns as intense – clear – radiance from within.

With unconstrained presence that neither "is" nor "is not",
Here, we look directly at defocused sensory appearance,
Here, because we rest naturally in ungraspable space,
Here, subliminal value judgment vanishes without trace,
And here, unfixed experience wells up from within.
This, simply, is the guru-vision matrix in the vastness of the now.

In the same way, when we are desirous and joyously fulfilled
By easy success, friends, good news, pleasure in wealth,
And by places and vistas, such pleasure enriches the mind with joy.
Recognize this, and naturally disposed, freely resting,
Uncontrived spontaneity occurs in pristine spaciousness.

When a neutral state of unaffected indifference possesses us,
No matter what arises, neither pleasant nor unpleasant,
Recognize it at its inception, without repression or indulgence,
And it falls into its own naturally disposed reality
Where neither differentiation nor exclusion impinges:
And "dullness is released into the sublime clear light".

At night, or whenever sleep overtakes us,
Lying down, naturally disposed, free from mental pulsation,
Gross appearances have subsided and with them our attachment.
When attachment to the subtle and very subtle has also vanished,
The mind as pure presence in its aspect of unthinking sameness
Abides in its own nature, free of the aberrations of hope and fear.
At this time all basic thought constructs are released as intrinsic
    spaciousness,
And it is described as "the release of samsara into nirvana".

As in sleep, so in the self-sprung pristine supermatrix,
Creative expressions dissolve into essential basic spaciousness
And all the elaboration perceived there as display subsides by itself.
In guru-vision, such is the involuntary function of self-sprung
    awareness.

In that way all desirable, undesirable and neutral mental states,
The three poisons,[30] arise in creativity as display,
Emerging from intrinsic spaciousness as spaciousness,
And since that includes everything, nothing excepted,
Nothing ever moves an iota from intrinsic spaciousness.
Avoiding anticipation and manipulation of it,
The recognition of spaciousness itself, and resting therein, is crucial
For thereby it naturally subsides, vanishing, released just as it is.

Afflictive emotion, karma and habitual propensities
Arise as illusory magical display from creativity,
And even methods of improvement on the path of liberation
Arise as illusory magical display from creativity:
Everything arises in the now as display of creativity
And it is crucial to recognize it without modifying it in any way.

All the same in posture, same in gait,
The same in relation to the ground,
Transcending circumstance, complexity and causality,
And causality superseded, resting freely,
We cherish our natural disposition.

This then is the peak of the supreme secret approach.
Do not speak of it to those of lesser acumen – keep it highly secret.
Interpretation will distort the heart teaching,
And exaggerated appreciation is at odds with the vision.
Violators of secrecy fall eternally into the lower realms,
So the legacy of this sovereign secret approach,
This teaching, is entrusted only to the fortunate fearless few.

*

In short, no matter what situation arises
Do not engage in it to improve it or to try to suppress it,
For the key is pure presence, naturally disposed, freely resting.

Pure presence may occur as pleasure or pain,
But if we discriminate between them
We are caught in conditioned existence.

Everything that appears in the sensory field is identical,
Just clarity in the face of the sense organ;
Everything that arises in the mind is identical,
Just the same traceless thought;
The juncture of object and mind is identical,
Just the same binding reaction pattern;
In truth, ultimately, every perception is identical,
Just groundless, baseless appearance;
Sensory objects all have an identical tendency,
Just traceless in their unraveling;
Mental states have an identical face,
Just space when identified;
Object and mind are nondual – just pure open space:
Whoever knows this is the heir of the All-Good,
The supreme bodhisattva, the highest vidhyadhara.

Therefore, all experience, equally absent, is identical,
Equally apparent and equally empty, equally true and equally false,
And we may dispense with all antidotes, all striving, all fixations,
And space out in objectless sameness;
Space out in mindless marvelous presence;
Space out in infallible superlative sameness.

Canto Twelve: Release

Introductory

In rational minds trained to ignore or reject "excluded middle" the imperative mood of the verb tends to invoke either defensive or enthusiastic response. Everyone who has been conditioned by an educational system designed to induce order, establish fixed categories and logical thinking, tends to react with one extreme or the other. Those who have been through a subsequent boot camp where thoughtful response is superseded by instinctual obedience may respond immediately and without consideration to direct commands. Obedience and moral sensitivity seem to be mutually exclusive. So, herein, in this translation and commentary, the imperative voice has been kept to a minimum, and even the hortative voice is sometimes softened. On occasion, however, an imperative can work like the syllable phat, like a wake-up call, like an explosion that clears the mind and frees the spirit. "Freedom" is the salient word here, for without emptying the mind, without recognizing the emptiness of the mind, we cannot recognize the natural process of release that is the equivalent of knowing the simultaneous traceless arising and dissolution of whatever arises into consciousness.

This freedom is coincident with nonaction. Nonaction is not to be understood merely as sitting still and remaining immobile for a given period. It is not a matter of keeping the voice and the energy of the bodymind silent and still. So long as the mind is conditioned to achieve goals predicated upon a set of principles or strictures or precepts, and habitually makes discriminating choices in order to attain those goals and remain faithful to principles, when the bodymind is set free from its formal session of meditation it will automatically revert to "action". The evidence of this action will be seen in the constancy of its preferences and bias, in its habitual cultivation of this and its renunciation of that, in its built-in likes and dislikes, in its endeavors and its questing. Nonaction, on the contrary, expresses itself as spontaneity, without any pattern or self-interested motivation, an uncontrived, involuntary responsiveness – or let's call it compassion.

The essence of this instruction upon release is the assertion of release as an automatic reflex of the creativity of pure presence. Unlike a soap bubble bursting adventitiously in the sky, unlike the process of dying when the extent of the lifespan has been reached, the apparent manifestation and release of creativity, are simultaneous – and thus it has no extension in time. For this reason it is said to "leave no residue". This momentary – or constant – release is imaged as a flight path of a bird in the sky. However, the reflexive process is inhibited by an absence of confidence in it. In other words, recognition is required in order for reflexive release to engage. Through the confidence that is able to let go of the habitual grasping at an object fixed in consciousness by the sensory process, the reflexive process is recognized. This confidence is engendered by experience of relaxation into the nature of mind. It may be coincident with nonaction and release or, perhaps, still present in the afterglow of initiatory experience. The confidence is strengthened by the snowball effect as familiarization with reflexive release grows.

In short, the function of a repressive and grasping mind in or through time is to reify each event, and believing that the event is real and concrete, to engage with it in a positive or negative frame and to perceive it accordingly as either good or bad. Collaterally, contriving a causal chain, unthinkingly or not, imagining – fabricating – a primary cause for the event and also a primary effect, the cause is the karmic residue from a previous event and the effect is the residue of this event that will be understood as the cause of a future event. Each event thus reinforces propensities that as an aggregation define our personality and samsaric fate. The "residue" becomes the bricks and mortar of karma with which a prison is built for us in one of the six mythic realms. The confidence inherent in nonaction and in the natural state of being that is precipitated in nonaction allows us to recognize the natural process of release. In that release habitual propensities of mind are uprooted, the maw of karma vanishes like the fading away of a Cheshire cat, karmic drive is exhausted – the winds of karma weaken, so that the suffering implied by birth is nullified and the body of light is facilitated.

The doubt that the intellect throws up in the absence of the confidence engendered in initiatory experience is always delusory. As the first stanza of this canto affirms and successive stanzas reaffirm, nothing in reality is not released; only in samsaric delusion does it appear that residue is left over from mental events. With confidence in release the karmically induced illusory visions of samsara are recognized first as the playful interactions of multi-colored star-dashed space and finally as the consummation of reality.

RELEASE

"All experience is released in the now in luminous mind."

All experience is released, here and now, in luminous mind –
An unreleased event is impossible.

Samsara is released in the now,
Liberated as alpha-purity;
Nirvana is released in the now,
Liberated as spontaneous perfection;
Appearances are released in the now,
Liberated in their baselessness;
Life is released in the now,
Liberated in its luminous heart;
Mental elaboration is released in the now,
Liberated in its limitlessness;
Formlessness is released in the now,
Liberated as pure potential.

Pleasure is released in the now,
Liberated in its equalized reality;
Suffering is released in the now,
Liberated in the ubiquitous basic expanse;
Dispassion is released in the now,
Liberated in the skylike dharmakaya;
Purity is released in the now,
Liberated in its empty authenticity;
Impurity is released in the now,
Liberated in supreme spacious freedom.

The levels and paths are released in the now,
Liberated in the absence of creative and fulfillment stages;
View and meditation are released in the now,
Liberated in nondiscrimination;
Conduct is released in the now,
Liberated in the All-Good;
The goal is released in the now,
Liberated in the absence of hope and fear;
Samayas are released in the now,
Liberated in the supreme reality;
Recitation is released in the now,
Liberated in nonverbal expression;
Contemplation is released in the now,
Liberated in the absence of a field of thought.

Affirmation and negation are released in the now,
Liberated in the middle way;
Dogmatic belief is released in the now,
Liberated in absence of any ground;
Authenticity is released in the now,
Liberated in absence of any preconception;
Inauthenticity is released in the now,
Liberated in noncritical bias;
Karma is released in the now,
Liberated in its boundless transparency;
Afflictive emotion is released in the now,
Liberated in thorough disinterest;
Karmic proclivity is released in the now,
Liberated in its groundlessness;
Karmic result is released in the now,
Liberated in the discontinuity of experience.

Antidotal method is already released,
Liberated in self-sufficiency,
Liberated in the vast skylike expanse of nondual give and take;
Catharsis is released in the now,
Liberated in nonrepression;
Repression is released in the now,
Liberated in skylike freedom;

Hanging loosely is released in the now,
Liberated by the absence of anything to relax;
Resting freely is released in the now,
Liberated by the absence of anything brought to rest.

*

In short, all conscious sensory perception,
And all that is unconscious or transcendent,
Everything is already released in the spaciousness of the now,
So any attempt to liberate anything anew is superfluous.

It is pointless to try to make effort towards release!
So don't try! Don't try! Don't struggle and strive in practice!
Don't seek! Don't seek! Don't seek intellectual truth!
Don't meditate! Don't meditate! Don't contrive meditation!
Don't analyze! Don't analyze! Don't analyze in or after an event!
Don't practice! Don't practice! Don't practice the upshot of hope
    and fear!
Don't reject! Don't reject! Don't reject emotional karma!
Don't believe! Don't believe! Don't believe in righteous religion!
Don't trap yourself! Don't trap yourself! Don't cage your mind!

In the absence of an objective field, everything equalized,
No discernable point of reference, no object and no order, can exist;
The ground collapses, the path collapses and the goal collapses,
And thoughts of good or bad, deviation and error, are inconceivable;
Committed to equalization, bound in the now, the universe resolved,
Samsara and nirvana have reverted to ubiquitous spaciousness.
The questions "What is it?" "How is it?" lie unanswered.
"What can I do?" "Who am I?" likewise, unanswerable!
What can we do when all our certainties have vanished?
We can only laugh outright at the absurdity of it.

The entire galaxy of delusory constructs, inner and outer, collapses
And linear time melts in the now, self-dissolving, fading into space;
Days and dates fade away; months, years and eons dissolve;
The one and the many vanished, sacred and profane both clarified;
The delusive ground of samsara and nirvana clarified in its innate
    spaciousness.

Even "spaciousness", as an intellectually contrived entity, dissolves.
Whatever we have practiced, however we strive, is useless now,
And intellectual gall exhausted, what a great marvel is the sky –
This pathless vagrant is one with the sky!

Since this floating jeweline sky-fortress, lacking foundation,
Released in the now, arises spontaneously as guru-vision,
The threefold universe is released as objectless sublimity.

                                        *

People consensually bound in delusory space-time,
Ignorant of their own intrinsic nature are corrupted
And stupefy themselves. Such delusion!
Their delusion lies in seeing the absence of delusion as an abyss.

Deluded or not, the same luminous-mind matrix pertains,
And there in the now, neither delusion nor release occurs.
Reification of what arises from luminous mind as display entraps us –
Both confinement and release are nondual, the mind and its field
        nonexistent!
Do not be seduced into believing that what is mere label truly exists!

Pure presence is liberated by buddha in the now,
So do not confine it in the trap of goal-fixation.
In the now, in the pure matrix of no objectivity,
In the luminous matrix that is blissful skylike root and base,
As alpha-purity, samsara is not possible.

Within the one sole sphere without edges or corners,
The deluded mind holds ideas of unity and differentiation;
Within the self-sprung awareness in the now without causes or
        conditions,
What holds to the samsaric process is a luminous obstructing spirit;
Within unlimited, nonspatial, spontaneity,
Attachment to a determinate view is the devil of conceit;
Within the noncrystallizing emptiness free of substance and attribute
Perverse intellect infers presence or absence, appearance or emptiness:

Abandon the cage of determinacy and bias
And know the nonspatial spontaneity that is like the sky!

Whatever arises in the six sensory fields, all sound and appearance,
All is intrinsic clarity in the undifferentiating, all-inclusive matrix:
Let us come to resolution in the now in that matrix of sameness.

Awareness as "spaciousness" gives rise to all appearance in unitary
     sameness;
Awareness as "the ground of being" generates all potential;
Awareness as "the matrix" liberates everything without any application;
Awareness as "luminous mind" is the essential universal source:
Know all things as pristine purity like the sky.[31]

Self-sprung awareness is the vast basic matrix of luminous mind:
Undefiled – untouched by samsara – it is luminous,
Uncaused – all potentiation as spontaneity it is luminous,
And as pure clear light – the heart of intrinsic presence – it is mind.
In luminous mind everything, all included, is completely pure.

With realization of the original face of what arises out of creativity as
     display,
A sudden reawakening to buddha may occur;
In the absence of realization, oblivious conditioned consciousness arises
In eight fields[32] of dualistic perception developed from a genetic basis,
And yet, however the resultant display of the universe appears,
It can never stray from the matrix of luminous mind,
And unmoving from the luminous mind matrix, staying in sameness,
Samsara and nirvana are united and released in the vast guru-vision
     matrix.

In the natural disposition, samsara and nirvana are impossible;
Goal-fixation is impossible in the natural disposition;
The five emotional syndromes are impossible in the natural disposition;
Fragmentation and partiality are impossible in the natural disposition;
Self-expression is impossible in the natural disposition:
In the natural disposition, nothing ever crystallizes.

With self-sprung awareness in the now, consummate in nameless reality,
No matter what arises, rootlessly, as creativity and display,
It falls naturally, without confinement or release, as natural perfection.
"Release" or "liberation" is cypher for "naturally dissolving without
   residue"
And since "everything exists" and "nothing exists" are not contradictory,
It is expressed by the words "released in the now".

No differentiation or exclusivity, just release in the matrix of
   spontaneity!
No union or separation, just release in the matrix of the one sole sphere!
No matter what manifests, it is released in the indeterminable matrix!

Manifest as form – shining, released just as it is!
Audible as sound – vibrating, released just as it is!
Perceptible as smell – released in its own spaciousness!
Savored as taste, felt as tactile sensations – released in its own space!
And thought, apprehended, groundless, unsupported, rootless
   – always released.

Liberation in unity – released in the matrix of reality!
Nonduality – released in the sameness of object and mind!
Self-sprung liberation – released in the matrix of primal awareness!
Spontaneous liberation – released in the pure spaciousness of the
   ground!

Multiplicity liberated – released as the one sole matrix!
Indeterminacy liberated – released as the spontaneity of the matrix!
Everything liberated – released as the heart-matrix!

The clear light released – liberated in the stellar matrix!
Reality released – liberated in the sky-matrix!
The objective field released – liberated in the oceanic matrix!
Unchanging release – liberation in the peak-matrix.

Released from the first – released in the matrix of potential!
Totality released – liberated in the matrix, buddha in the now!
Total release, release in the now – liberation in the constantly
   unfolding matrix!

Canto Thirteen: Buddha

Introductory

"Buddhahood" is the term used in the Buddhist sutras to describe the goal at the end of the Buddhist path. Buddhahood is a goal to be accomplished way down the path, beyond the horizon, certainly not in this lifetime, and probably only after eons of strenuous effort. The slightly pompous, far distant, entity worshipped in Thai temples, Vietnamese Zen shrines, Tibetan gompas and so on around the world embodies a transcendent principle of omniscience that moves people to devotion and prayer. This sanctimonious "Buddhahood" of the Buddhist religion is of no use in Dzogchen. In Dzogchen we are too close to the raw existential intensity of awareness and compassion; too close to the clarity and spontaneity of the clear light. We need a word that expresses the enlightenment inherent in the here and now. That word is simply "buddha", which implies such intimacy that we cannot separate ourselves from it. It is so close that no distance separates us and it. The "principle" is never a concept because in the now buddha is not objectified or reified. The root of the word "buddha" denotes cognition, not the cognition belonging to sensory consciousness, but to existential being in itself that is self-aware spaciousness. "Buddha" is thus a synonym of the light of the mind.

In Dzogchen, belief that Gautama, the son of a wealthy landowner in Northern India, attained enlightenment under the bodhi-tree in Bodhgaya is superfluous. Surely, belief in events happening in past, present or future lands tend to lead to reification of space-time. The events in the Indian country of Magadha twenty-five hundred years ago are as illusory as twentieth century events, no event having any greater significance than any other in so far as all events are figments of mind, insubstantial, evanescent, like rainbow-colored gossamer floating on the breeze. Belief in "significant events" occurring in space-time are distractions from the sameness of the blissful nondual experience of the here and now, says Longchenpa – although for him, of course, there can never be distraction. Even a moment's entrancement in the creativity of imagined mythical events that brought superlative kindness into a cruel world, however, is not separation from the nature of mind in which it manifests.

Following an exposition of the inseparable view and meditation of Dzogchen, it is quite usual to find a teaching on the bardos attached. Instruction on the bardos is like an addendum to the root Dzogchen precepts. It has already been said that when the karmic propensities of embodiment have been clarified, or once they have dissolved, only the rainbow body remains. Now, the same principal is applied to the mode of being at death and immediately thereafter. Here the simile of the garuda's birth is evoked. The great garuda bird, the mythic Himalayan eagle, is said to mature fully within the egg. When it hatches and the egg breaks open, the garuda immediately spreads its wings and from the high crag where lies his aerie soars into the sky. Likewise, when the concrete shell of embodiment cracks open and shatters at the moment of death, like space meeting space when a door is opened, dissolution into self-aware spaciousness occurs and buddha is synchronistically revealed. The simile of the garuda's birth may illustrate the occurrence at the moment of death; but the bardo of dying is a metaphor for the manner of release from embodiment during the bardo of life. It is surely the fear that possesses anxious, miserable people in the maw of death, clutching at straws in their trepidation, which allows them to interpret the bardo teaching and the bardo visions as premonition of an afterlife. To withdraw that hope from them is like refusing a drink of water to a dying man, but the kindness of providing it is an excellent excuse to veil the knowledge of radical Dzogchen.

BUDDHA

"Free of all striving and endeavor, all experience in luminous mind is
    buddha."

If we gain familiarity with the luminous essence,
The luminous spontaneity of things,

Through the key precepts of nonstriving and effortlessness,
Buddha in the now is buddha reawakened
And that is the actuality of the peerless vajra-heart,
The essence of the ninefold path, the luminous supermatrix.

The sun and moon – clear light mandalas – in the vault of the sky,
Obscured by thick clouds, are invisible:
Just so, the luminosity within us is veiled.

Just as thick clouds floating in the sky may naturally disperse,
So the miasma of causality involuntarily dissolves by itself,
And the luminous heart arises by itself in the vault of the sky.
But different degrees of acumen require different approaches.

Our original face shines like the sun in the matrix of intrinsic
     spaciousness,
Its creativity, without bias, projecting everything as light,
Filling the land and the oceans with warmth,
So that moisture arises as a cloud display
That seems to veil our essence and our creativity besides.
An impure display of essence and creativity
Veils the original face of reality that is our heart-essence
Covering it with a universe of incalculable delusive appearances.

Out of creative power a wind blows,
And similar to the sun's rays, it disperses the clouds;
As we realize our original face,
The display is experienced as ornamentation;
Delusion, released in the now, is now liberated as it stands,
And deluded perception and attachment, without denunciation,
Lie at peace, assuaged in their own spaciousness.

The great garuda's wings develop within the egg,
But enveloped by the shell this is not apparent;
When it hatches, instantly, it soars into the sky.
Likewise, although delusive dualistic perception is already resolved,
Only when the shell of congealed residue cracks open
Does the intrinsically clear spontaneity of pure presence arise by itself.
Manifestations of buddha in buddhafields fill the spacious sky,

And through recognition of the original face
We are liberated in the all-good matrix.

*

As a boundless display of compassion filling the ten directions,
Miraculous emanation satisfies the needs of beings;
For as long as samsara lasts such altruistic activity flourishes,
Activity that arises out of the naturally settled essence of being
As display of our creativity's impartial compassion
Abundantly benefitting others.

Impure display has completely collapsed,
Yet transforming emanation suffuses impure beings
By means of the teacher's appropriate responsiveness
And by open-minded people's pure aspiration.

Presently, although incalculable environments exist,
Countless beings therein being drawn into luminosity,
They cannot stray from the spaciousness of the teachers' dharmakaya,
For self-sprung awareness is unrestricted – zero-dimensional.
Naturally occurring within spaciousness as the highest envisionment[33]
An inconceivable sambhogakaya array manifests
To fearless, tenth-level rigzin and dakinis.
It is as if, through the teacher's spacious compassion,
And the disciple's devotion and virtue,
Mind's original face surely shines forth as spontaneity.

In this self-sprung awareness in the now, itself the dharmakaya,
The all-inclusive display is a lake of all-knowing impartial awareness,
The one sole sphere of pristine spaciousness.

The essence of the sambhogakaya is natural spontaneity,
And the five buddha-families and the five modes of primal awareness
As display of pure presence, fill the entire gamut of the sky.

The essence of the nirmanakaya is the ground of manifest compassion,
The display appearing wherever and as whatever action is needed,
Demonstrating thereby perfectly appropriate activity.

These modes of being defy goal-directed endeavor;
They shine only in freely resting space as the spontaneity of the now.
This supreme secret is disclosing itself at this moment,
And since we shall not be lured away from it, even in the bardo,
This apex approach of the vajra-heart,
Towers, exalted, above all progressive, graduated approaches.

Conclusion

This song of the vajra-heart of reality,
Its alpha-pure nature like the sky,
Occurs as a self-arisen display
Neither transforming nor sublimating
In unchanging groundless space.

It evokes the vast supermatrix, the all-pervasive sameness of the now,
So that without going anywhere, in the natural state of alpha-purity,
In unrestricted and zero-dimensional freedom,
We may enter the reality of immutable spontaneity.

The center of the vast skylike expanse is our concern,
The sovereign self-sprung supermatrix,
Where, unmoving, everything is released as its stands,
Where we reach the vast womb of ineffable spaciousness.

Such a skylike adept, his realization certain,
Composed this short poem from his own experience
In accordance with the formal transmission and the scriptures –
The twenty-one texts of the mind series,
The three sections of the matrix series
And the four sections of the secret precept series.

Through the merit of this work may all beings, excluding none,
Without effort, realize the space of alpha-purity,
And as princes of reality spontaneously provide mutual benefit
In the unalterable, nonsublimating, realm of Samantabhadra.

Let comfort and ease and prosperity spread everywhere
And as in a pure land, may wishes be spontaneously fulfilled;
As the drum of reality beats, the banner of freedom unfurled,
Fearless awareness is sustained and Dzogchen revelation increases.

An adept of the apex approach, Longchen Rabjampa, composed this Treasury of the Dharmadhatu *in the throat of the White Skull Snow Mountain and it is now completed.*

Notes to the Text

1   The three dimension of being; the three buddha bodies.
2   The mythic realms of gods, men, demons, hungry ghosts, animals and hell-beings.
3   Womb, egg, moisture and miraculous birth.
4   The five external sensory fields and the mental field.
5   *Sku dang ye shes*. See *Notes*: Buddha in buddhafields.
6   *Tshogs chen*.
7   *Srid gsum*: past, present and future.
8   *Gzer chen gsum: dpe don rtags*: similitude, evocation and evidence.
9   The root text has "without distinction between past, present and future".
10 The commentary provides *rtogs dang mi rtogs* (realized or unrealized).
11 *Spyi blugs:* empowerment by libation as in a Hindustani prince's investiture.
12 *Khams gsum*: sensual, aesthetic and formless realms.
13 '*Char nub rnyog pa*; also *spro 'dus pa.*
14 *Dbye bsal (gsal) med pa*: without differentiation or exclusion; "without sharpness or blur" is a togal interpretation.
15 *Zang thal.*
16 A holographic mirror.
17 *Rang bzhin bcu*, the ten tantric constituents: view, meditation, conduct, goal, stages and paths,mandala, mantra, fulfillment stage, empowerment, samaya.
18 Sravaka, pratyekabuddha and bodhisattva approaches.
19 *Byang chub gsum*: three levels of effulgence.
20 *Nyon mongs lnga*: desire, anger, pride, jealousy and stupidity.

21 *Gnam gzer*: mainstay, kingpin; "a lock of spaciousness".

22 *Klu:* subterranean serpent spirits of mother earth.

23 *Phyal ba lhug pa gzhi med zang ka ma:*
   Gtad med zang zing ban bun chal ma chol.

24 Klong chen rab 'byams: Longchenpa's formal name.

25 Sna tshogs rang grol: Natsok Rangdrol, one of Longchenpa's personal names.

26 Klong chen rab 'byams pa.

27 Cardinal and intermediate directions, zenith and nadir.

28 *Zhi gnas:* shamata meditation.

29 *Kun yin kun min yin min*: "beyond positivism and nihilism, beyond is and is not".

30 *Dug gsum:* lust, hatred and sloth.

31 The commentary's addition of *ye shes* "awareness in the now" as the topic of this stanza makes best sense.

32 The eight fields of perception are the fields of the five external senses plus the internal fields of thought, emotion and the ground of being.

33 *Stug po bkod pa*, or *'Og min*, the Akanishta Paradise.

Appendix 1

A List of Similes and Metaphors

NB The text contains thirty-seven instances of the adjective "skylike" or the adjectival phrase "like the sky" applied variously to reality, spaciousness, matrix, supermatrix, dharmakaya, pure presence, nature of mind, path, vision, adept, illusion, situations etc., most of which have been omitted in this list to avoid repetition.

Canto One

The nature of mind is an unchanging, skylike supermatrix...

And the six fields[34] of dualistic sense perception of the universe,
Appearing in their own spaciousness, like magical illusion, do not
    truly exist...

Already arrived, nothing to do, without any practice,
Like the sun in the sky – that is an amazing, superb reality.

Here in this womb-like spaciousness, in the spontaneity of the now,
Samsara is all good...

And pure like the sky, nothing can ever be restricted or localized:
That is alpha-pure vision of ultimate liberation.

Canto Two

As pure presence, it is clear like the sky, nonspatial, nondual;
As the vast matrix itself, it is beyond pulsating thought and image.

All the phantasmagoria of life and death, pleasure and pain,
Like apparitional show, abounds in the matrix of mind in itself...

Apparent, yet insubstantial and hence truly nonexistent,
It occurs through adventitious circumstance,
Like moisture condensing as clouds...

The nature of mind, the essential luminous mind,
Pure like the sky, free of birth and death, pleasure and pain...

Within that palace arrayed with spontaneously amassed wealth,
The king Self-sprung Awareness takes his throne;
His pulsated projections, the creations of his pristine awareness,
Serve as ministers who govern his domain;
The holy queen Innate Meditative Absorption attends,
With Spontaneous Guru-Vision, her offspring, and her servants,
All centered in the pure pleasure matrix of intrinsic, nonconceptual
    clarity.

Canto Three
The simile for luminous mind is "skylike".

Luminous mind is like the solar nucleus:
Its nature is clear light, forever uncompounded...

Things appear but they never crystallize:
Everything is like mirage, dream, echo,
Like apparition, reflection in water and castles in the sky.
Like hallucination, things are clearly apparent, but do not truly exist.

Pure presence, unbreakable, is the luminous matrix;
Skylike spaciousness, unalterable and unchangeable, saturates the
    now...

People's unrealized strobe-like perception in the mundane world...

Canto Five

We know that reality itself, like the sun,
Stays forever in its natural state of all-embracing clear light...

Canto Six

Just as all sunlight is considered the nature of the sun,
So all experience is the nature of luminous mind.

All of it noncomposite, empty clarity, like sun-dashed space,
All of it the vast, pristine, self-sprung matrix of the now.

The vast matrix of mind's nature, an unchanging skylike space,
With the creativity of luminous mind indeterminate in its display,
Governs all the lifestyles of samsara and nirvana,

Like an emperor magisterially embodying the state
The entirety of samsara and nirvana is governed unmoving.

Canto Seven

And the matrix of immaculate intrinsic presence is like that –
Like water when the sediment has settled, natural purity revealed.

Canto Eight

Without body, object or perception as a reference point,
Our all-pervasive smoothness the same as the vast expanse of the sky...

The dharmakaya citadel naturally arises within our inner nature,
And it is immaculate – "Like the sky!" we say,
Although it is actually incommensurable.

Canto Nine

In the one sole sphere the linear, causal, process is reversed,
And skylike sameness unravels goal-related hope and fear.
It is vast, it is magnificent – skylike buddha-mind!
Without goal-fixation – the matrix of the one sole sphere!
Liberation in the now – whether or not we are realized!
Happy the yogin on the skylike path of nonaction!

Canto Ten
This is the vajra-peak, the supreme all-good buddha-mind,
The most sublime spacious event, as high as the sky.

Crystal clear space, free of alternation and pulsation,
Like a still, unsullied, translucent ocean,

Everything dissolving is released in the now,
And its nature is like the sky.

Hanging loose, like someone who has nothing to lose,
Neither tense nor slack, the bodymind rests comfortably.

Although the matrix is thoughtfree and spacious like the sky,
We are caught in a cage of reified concepts.

Canto Eleven
"All situations are pure like the sky

Within the unitary luminous mind where everything is the same as
    the sky,
Dualistic perception deludes us with causal, conditioned existence...

Canto Twelve
Abandon the cage of determinacy and bias
And know the nonspatial spontaneity that is like the sky!

Know all things as pristine purity like the sky.

Canto Thirteen
Our original face shines like the sun in the matrix of intrinsic
    spaciousness,

The sun and moon – clear light mandalas – in the vault of the sky,
Obscured by thick clouds, are invisible:
Just so, the luminosity within us is veiled.

Just as thick clouds floating in the sky may naturally disperse,
So the miasma of causality involuntarily dissolves by itself...

Concluding Verses

And as princes of reality spontaneously provide mutual benefit
In the unalterable, unsublimating, realm of Samantabhadra.

Appendix 2

Notes on the Translation and Technical Vocabulary of *Radical Dzogchen*

Generally, the Tibetan root text is well edited and reliable. Sometimes, however, poor calligraphy has led to creeping errors that have been corrected in the commentary (e.g. *klong* to *blo* in canto 9, verse 6, and verse 9). Sometimes the commentary has a phrase that I have preferred over the root text simply by subjective bias: *gnyis su med* to *byar med shing* (canto 10, verse 33) and *rgya chad* to *rtag chad* (canto 13, verse 6).

Where versification requires it, I have made one line into two. I have added asterisks sometimes to break up the cantos into integral sections, sometimes, it may seem, quite arbitrarily, to aid the reader's comprehension. In a few places where the imperative mood of the verb seemed too demanding, too challenging, I have moderated it. I have followed the Tibetan construction with "non" for *med* too much for poetic tolerance.

These notes on the vocabulary of radical Dzogchen include the reasons for choosing the English phrase to render a specific Tibetan phrase. They are organized in English alphabetic order. Tibetan phrases in this section are also included in the following section, *Appendix 3: Tibetan-English Dzogchen Wordlist*, where they are organized in Tibetan alphabetic order.

All-pervasive smoothness, *phyam gdal*

The difficult word *phyam* and its compounds remain without definitive English equivalents. More applicable in the togal context, *phyam 'dal* indicates experience that has been equalized and thus constitutes a smoothed-out space, a uniform space informing multiplicity, a space of complexity unraveled and thus assumes a reality in which appearances have been homogenized yet somehow retain their specificity. Thus *phyam gcig* is sometimes rendered "totality". *Phyam 'dal* also lends itself to translation as "a pixelated field". Richard Barron has rendered it "infinite evenness".

Buddha, *sang rgyas*

"Buddha" (*sang rgyas*) in the Hinayana and Mahayana contexts is a personification of nonduality or of a supposed attribute of nonduality. This personification, or anthropomorphism, perhaps serves a didactic purpose in devotional Buddhism, but in Dzogchen it obscures the impersonal, nondual reality. I have avoided therefore both definite and indefinite articles. "Buddha" has no attribute, no person, no specific. "Simple recognition of the nature of being is labeled 'buddha'" (canto 10, verse 20).

Buddha in buddhafields, *sku dang ye shes*

The phrase *sku dang ye shes* denotes Dzogchen reality by juxtaposing two nondual terms, *sku* meaning buddha-body or buddha-dimensionality, or sublime form, and *ye shes* denoting awareness in the now, primal or primordial awareness, or alpha-pure or pristine awareness. Placing them together creates a phrase denoting both ontic and epistemic ultimacy. "Immaculate being and awareness in the now" is a fairly literal translation; herein I have used "buddha in buddhafields", the more poetical equivalent.

Confinement, *bcings, ma grol ba*

The antonym of release or liberation could be confinement, captivity, or bind or bondage. Sometimes I have rendered *bcings* as repression.

Contemplation, *ting nge 'dzin*

Although *bsam gtan* and *ting nge 'dzin* are often interchangeable, the first is usually the meditative concentration of the graduated path and the second the contemplation of nonmeditation.

Dualistic perception, *bzung 'dzin*

Bzung 'dzin is often translated as "dualistic perception", *bzung* referring to the objective element and *'dzin* to the subjective knower that grasps an object. What is held in that situation of dualistic perception is automatically reified and what grasps at and is attached to any object of perception is also reified, even as it reifies the object of its perceiving. The notion of reification, or rather the notion absence of reification, is vital in the noncrystallizing process of the emanation and dissolution of creativity within luminous mind.

Essence/nature, *ngo bo, rang bzhin*

Whereas in the context of the trikaya I have translated *ngo bo* and *rang bzhin* as "essence" and "nature" respectively, where *ngo bo* appears in the conjunction of *ye shes* and *rol pa,* for instance, I have translated it as "nature", and where *rang bzhin* points at something "inner", I have sometimes rendered it as "essential".

Experience, *chos*

A case exists for reconsideration of the English equivalent of *chos* in Dzogchen contexts. In the abhidharma, or mainstream Buddhist metapsychology, *dharma* or *chos* in its technical sense is generally translated as "phenomena". "Phenomena" is understood as external appearances, although from the point of view of Mind Only it may refer to the phenomena of mind and therefore signify internal events. In either case, "phenomena" implies an objective reference. In Dzogchen "phenomena" as an objective reference is the product of a delusive function of the relative mind, implying karmic attachment. In Dzogchen, what in the lower approaches, in a dualistic view, is denominated "phenomena" must be reviewed in the unitary light of the dharmadhatu. The English word that may mean whatever arises, or does not arise, is simply "experience". All "experience" is the nondual phenomena of perception, where subject and object and inner and outer and mind and its objects are an inseparable unity. Thus, "experience" is dharma and intrinsic spaciousness (dharmadhatu) is the intrinsic nature of all experience.

Luminous mind, *byang chub sems*, bodhichitta

A strong case can be presented for assimilating the word *bodhichitta*, by which we understand compassionate buddha mind, into the English language – we possess no equivalent. "Enlightened mind" or "awakened mind" is the phrase most commonly employed as its equivalent in the Vajrayana. But in the Vajrayana, enlightened mind is the prerogative of a Buddha or Bodhisattva, whereas in Dzogchen it is the very stuff of all-embracing reality. The nondual imperative of Dzogchen requires a more neutral, less affective equivalent for bodhichitta, and for that reason I have chosen *luminous mind*, the luminous mind that supersedes or transcends the rational mind without any sense of moral quality. Mind is luminous under all circumstances, not only when the mind is awakened from delusion or when its darkness is enlightened on a progressive path. This bodhichitta – Mind - by definition is light, the clear light (*'od gsal*) synonymous with *rig pa*. Bodhichitta is the nature of mind (*sems nyid*). Luminous mind is also the sole recourse of beings trapped on a causal path, because it is the one cause and the sole effect. Luminous mind, however, is also identified as loving-kindness and selfless compassion.

Nonaction, *byar med*, *bya bral*

This term presents us with a similar koan-like paradox as *rigpa* qualified as immutable and unchangeable and the same paradox when reality (*chos nyid*) is qualified as sameness. "Free from activity" or "action" may provide a clue but does not give us the opportunity to resolve the paradox intuitively. In *The Divine Madman* I translated *byar med* as "duty-free" and in *Original Perfection* ("Great Garuda") as *bya bral* and "free-form action", but these are special cases and those terms cannot be used invariably. Insofar as nonaction implies "the action of nonaction", "nondeliberate" or "nondirected action" admits only half the story. Nonaction or non-doing is how Taoist translators conventionally render *wu wei*. The literal translation may not be poetic, but it is the only one that works here, I think, and besides constitutes a koan-like precept in itself.

Nonspatial and nontemporal, *phyogs ris med pa*

The Tibetan word *phyogs* denotes space and spatiality and, also, secondarily, mass or volume. *Phyogs med* or the absence of space indicates the zero dimension and, thus, adjectivally can be translated as "nondimensional", "nonspatial", or "nondirectional". *Phyogs med* can also mean "impartial", or "unbiased" and is thus a synonym of *ris med*, which, however, insofar as discrimination and bias imply an extension in time where two things may or may not be compared, signifies a nontemporal state. Thus, *phyogs ris med pa* may be rendered as "nonspatial and nontemporal".

Pristine, *gdod ma'i*

In general I have rendered *gdod ma'i* as "pristine" rather than the overworked and misleading "primordial". *Gdod nas* is still sometimes "primordially", however. Also, please note that *gdod nas* is a close synonym of *ka dag*.

Pulsation, *spro bsdu*

The compound word *spro bsdu* refers to the emanation of "display" (*rol pa*) out of (or, better, within) luminous mind (*byang chub sems*) through its creative power (*rtsal*), and its dissolution back into that luminous mind, yet not having left it. The "projection and dissolution" of thought (and also feeling and all sensory consciousness) is simultaneous, and yet there is an undeniable moment of appearance and at the same time a sense of the spaciousness out of which it arises (the paradox of unitary relative and ultimate truth). It is as if the mind were pulsating – and thus "pulsation".

Pure presence, *rig pa*

In this translation, I have used "pure presence" as the English equivalent of *rig pa* and "(primal or pristine) awareness in the now" for *ye shes*. "Intrinsic awareness" is a good equivalent of *rig pa* but it induces a notion of an extrinsic awareness. *Presence (of mind?)* is close to the notion of "attention", which is the meaning of *rig pa* in common usage.

Reality, *chos nyid*

Chos nyid is conventionally translated as "the true nature of phenomena", "ultimate nature" or some such similar phrase, in Dzogchen texts. This phrase tends to propel the reader into an analytic, abhidharma frame of mind, implying a dualistic state of consciousness, when what is indicated is the nondual nature of ordinary experience of the here and now that is best simply termed "reality". Likewise, in the Dzogchen context, *chos* (*dharma*) is sometimes "nondual experience" rather than "mental event" (or "religion" or "the teaching").

Release/liberation *grol ba*

The Tibetan word *grol ba* is very commonly used and not always in the context of liberation from the round of rebirth. In the psychological context, it can be rendered as "release", "free" or "liberate". I have chosen "release", where its meaning may be construed as release as of repressed trauma or fixated concept or any aspect of mind, or indeed the intellect itself. I have used "liberation" as a more overarching concept or as a second choice.

Resolution, *la zla ba*

If "a decisive experience", an alternative rendering, evokes a mystical experience of light and sound, it may be misleading as a translation of *la zla ba,* which signifies an indescribable experience, although "bliss", "nonthought" and "clarity" are best used to denominate it. Although such a decisive experience will be a moment to remember, the resolution of duality is not necessarily an experience with signs.

Space, *ngang*

The Tibetan language requires a spatial context for substantive abstractions, a requirement that is fulfilled by the word *ngang*, which can be translated by "state" or "realm". English does not need this crutch and I have generally omitted translation of *ngang*, although sometimes it has been translated by "space", as in the usage of the psychedelic subculture. The word "state", never appropriate when referring to *rig pa,* generally evokes the notion of a fixed state, a trance state, a samsaric fixation and, moreover, tends to reify the attribute. "The view is without basis and meditation is not a 'state'" (canto 9, verse 23).

Spaciousness, dharmadhatu, *chos dbyings*

The Sanskrit word *dharmadhatu*, the Tibetan *chos dbyings* of the title of this poem, should enter the English language, as no generally accepted equivalent has been coined. Literally, it means the "sphere of dharma", "the sphere of reality". I have used "spaciousness" or "intrinsic spaciousness" herein as English equivalents, because in the Dzogchen context we strive to induce an existential and experiential ambience. "Basic space", as an option, appears to me too concrete an attribute easily lending itself to reification – as Longchenpa asserts, the dharmadhatu does not actually exist.

Sphere/pixel, *thig le*

In the context of this explication of the dharmadhatu, as a synonym of dharmadhatu *thig le* is translated as "sphere" and *thig le gcig* and *thig le nyag gcig,* all synonyms, as "the one sole sphere". However, particularly in the togal context, *thig-le* can well be translated as "pixel".

Spontaneity *lhun grub*

I have tried to maintain the translation of *lhun grub* as "spontaneity" rather than use the clumsy and often ill-suited "spontaneous presence". The word "spontaneity", however, invites confusion with "instinctual", thereby adulterating sublime meaning with a feral signification. However, I have found no better word than spontaneity to describe the absence of any causal base in time or space for the awareness of *rig pa,* for in direct experience it is known neither as a continuum nor as a series of nano-instants. For the phrase *lhun mnyam,* "unremitting sameness" has been preferred to "spontaneous sameness", and usually the phrase *lhun rdzogs* is rendered as "spontaneous perfection".

Sublime form, *kaya, sku (trikaya, sku gsum)*

In this exposition of Longchenpa, the word *sku (kaya)* only appears in the word *sku gsum (trikaya),* where dharmakaya, sambhogakaya and nirmanakaya are indicated. These three kayas are three aspects of a single experientially indivisible, ineffable, reality of being. The exception is in the phrase *rdo rje snying po'i sku,* denominating the *kaya* of the vajra-heart, and although "dimension" could be used here, perhaps "sublime form" is a better equivalent. As an element of "*trikaya*", *kaya* may be translated as "dimension", but in the context of the bardos and in togal it is inadequate. Thus employing "the three dimensions" is a manner of labeling aspects of unitary reality; reality is uni-dimensional or zero-dimensional, depending upon which way it is approached.

Synchronicity, *rten 'grel*

A synchronicitous event is a nondual, luminous event free of cause and condition; an affinity to the experience of synchronicity as defined in Jungian psychology is assumed. "Synchronicity" in the Jungian context is experience of two or more events that are apparently causally unrelated or unlikely to occur together by chance, yet are experienced as occurring together in a meaningful manner.

The now, *ye, ye nas*

The little word *ye* peppers Dzogchen texts and is often ignored. If it is translated as "timeless", we have "timeless awareness" or "timeless matrix", which allows easy reification. But "Ye!" like "Eh!" is an onomatopoeic evocation of the now and can be translated as such: "awareness in the now" for *ye shes* and "matrix of the now" for *ye klong. Ye nas* is "in the here and now" rather than "primordially" (Jurassic or Devonian?!) or "originally" (at the time of the Big Bang?!).

Trekcho and togal, *'khregs bcod dang thod rgal*

The terms trekcho (*'khregs bcod*) and togal (*thod rgal*) appear once each in the text, neither of them used in the sense of stages on a graduated Dzogchen path. Rather trekcho means identifying with the nature of mind in every moment and togal means jumping fearlessly into the moment.

Universe, galaxy (dualistic world) *snang srid, snod bcud*

Two distinct Tibetan terms denote the appearances of the dualistic world. The first is *snang srid* that can be rendered as "appearances and possibilities" or "inanimate and animate". The second is *snod bcud*, "the container and the contents", "the inanimate and animate universe", "material and spiritual dimensions" or poetically "the chalice and the grail". Sometimes these two phrases are joined together; singularly or together, they indicate our universe.

View, *lta ba*

The Tibetan *lta ba* is always rendered as "view" in conformity with the conventional usage in Buddhist philosophy, where it is an intellectual perspective (*darshana*) upon reality. In Dzogchen, since "the view" is also the meditation, definitively no intellectual element is contained in this consummate view, and the view is nondual and spontaneous and always the same.

Vision, *dgongs pa*

The word "vision" appears in two senses, which should not be interchanged. The first sense is found in the translation of *dgongs pa*, which until this translation I have rendered as "enlightened intent" – "buddha-intentionality". Tulku Thondup showed me that the best sense of "vision" – signifying what we "see" in the moment as the ideal (the great perfection) – is the precise meaning of *dgongs pa*. Where the context does not explicate that meaning as a synonym of Dzogchen, I have added the descriptive word "guru" to "vision". The second sense is the translation of *snang ba,* which means "appearance" or "envisionment" as in *snang bzhi,* the four visions, where the first is a flash of *dgongs pa* and the last its fulfillment.

Within, *las*

Whereas in Tibetan "emanation" can only arise "out of" the spaciousness of the dharmadhatu, in English we can say that it arises "in" or "within" that spaciousness and thereby add an imputation of transcendence that is generally assumed in the Tibetan. Likewise "display" arises "within" creativity rather that "out of" it.

Without effort or practice, *rtsol sgrub med*

Rtsol sgrub means "striving-practice" and thus "endeavor" and "quest"; *rgyu 'bras rtsol sgrub* means "goal-directed endeavor". *Rtsol sgrub med* means "without effort or practice" and in Dzogchen implies an absence of any achievement or attainment inherent in a goal.

Appendix 3

A Tibetan-English Dzogchen Word List

In this glossary, the first word in the column of English equivalents is usually – not always – the best. The following words are synonyms of the first, or alternative translations of the Tibetan. The words in square brackets are conventional translations generally inappropriate in a Dzogchen text. Richard Barron's sometimes excellent choices are indicated by RB.

This glossary includes all the Tibetan phrases discussed in the previous appendix, *Appendix 2: Notes on the Translation and Technical Vocabulary of Radical Dzogchen*; these phrases are indicated by "See *Notes*: 'equivalent English phrase'".

ka dag	alpha-pure
kun khyab	all-pervading, all-encompassing
kun khyab gdal	all-pervading ~uniformity ~smoothness
kun rtog	habitual assumptions, thought patterns [preconceptions]
kun 'dus	all-inclusive, gathered, unified, included, subsumed
klong	matrix [expanse]
klong chen	supermatrix [vast expanse]
klong yangs	vast matrix
rkyen snang	circumstantial~ adventitious~ appearances; situations
sku	sublime form, kaya. See also *Notes*: Sublime form
sku gsum	trikaya, three dimensions of being
sku dang ye shes	buddha in buddhafields; "immaculate pure being and primal awareness of the now". See also *Notes*: Buddha in buddhafields
'khregs bcod	See *Notes*: Trekcho and togal
dgag sgrub	judgmental; value judgment; suppress or indulge, assertion or negation

dgongs pa	vision, guru-vision [enlightened intent RB]. See also *Notes*: Vision
gyin 'dar	unaffected, ingenuous [unfeigned RB]
grub pa	substantiated, actualized, perfected [ensured RB]
grol ba	release, liberation, freedom. See also *Notes*: Release/liberation
glod pa	hanging loose, relaxed [carefree]
glo bur	adventitious (like clouds condensing in the sky) [circumstantial, chance]
dgongs pa	vision, guru-vision [enlightened intent]. See also *Notes*: Vision
'gyu 'phro rtog	movement or proliferation of thought
'gro 'ong med	without ~coming or going, ~intercourse; unvarying
rgya chad phyogs lhung med pa unrestricted or localized, [unfragmented, unconfined]
rgya chad med	without ~limitation, ~parameters; boundless
rgya yan	uninhibited, unbounded, carefree
sgrims glod med	neither tense nor loose
brgyan pa	enriched
ngang	See *Notes*: Space
ngang bzhag	at rest ["staying in the state", fixed state]
nges med	indeterminate, uncertain, unpredictable, variable
ngo sprod	direct introduction, pointing out
ngo bo	See *Notes*: Essence/nature
dngos po'i mtshan ma concrete attribute
car phog tu	direct experience
cog gzhag	freely resting
bcings pa	bind, bondage See also *Notes*: Confinement
cho 'phrul	magical emanation
chos	See *Notes*: Experience
chos nyid	See *Notes*: Reality
chos dbyings	See *Notes*: Spaciousness
chig chod	immediacy; instantly [unique RB]
'jur bu	habitual compulsion
nyag gcig	the one sole...
gnyen po	antidote, method, curative method
gnyug ma	genuine, authentic
ting nge 'dzin	See *Notes*: Contemplation
gtad med	without reference
gtad 'dzin	goal-orientation [fixed construct RB]
btang gzhag	accept or reject, discrimination; expunge or espouse, discard or adopt, unwanted or embraced
rtag chad	affirmation and denial, dogmatic belief
rten 'grel	See *Notes*: Synchronicity
lta ba	See *Notes*: View
brtags	imputation
tha snyad	conventional designation
thad drang du	straight, direct
thig le	sphere, pixel, lightseed. See also *Notes*: Sphere/pixel
thig le nyag gcig	the one sole sphere
thig le chen po	all-embracing cosmic seed, maha-pixel
thug phrad	direct encounter

thod rgal	See *Notes*: Trekcho and Togal
gdal ba	smooth out, equalize, [fulfill, suffuse, saturate]
gdod ma'i	pristine. See also *Notes*: Pristine
gdod nas	original [primordial] [syn. ka dag]
'du 'phro	pulsating (projections), alternate projection and absorption [proliferation and re-absorption] [see also 'phro 'dus, spro bsdu]
'du 'bral med pa	neither doable not undoable, without union or separation
'dus pa	concentrated [subsumed RB]
dran pa	thought, recollection, memory
nam mkha'	sky, space
rnal ma	genuine
snang ba	appearance, phenomena, vision
snang srid	See *Notes*: Universe, Galaxy (dualistic world)
snod bcud	See *Notes*: Universe, Galaxy (dualistic world)
spang blang	refusal or approval, discriminate
spangs thob	moral preference [renunciation and attainment]
spyi blugs	empowering, investing; immediate saturating empowerment [omnipresent RB]
spro bsdu	mental pulsation, fluctuation [RB elaborations]. See also *Notes*: Pulsation
spro bsdu med	without ~alternate projection and absorption, ~introversion and extroversion [without aversion or yearning, ~positive or negative energy patterns]
sprod	(mental) elaboration (involved in the four extremes)
sprod med	unelaborated, simple
'pho 'gyur med pa	without alteration or sublimation [transition or change]
phyam	smooth, total, uniform [evenness RB]
phyam gcig	totality, a single all-encompassing pixel, common denominator [single state of evenness RB]; [syn. thig le gcig]
phyam mnyam	smoothed out, equal
phyam gdal	an all-pervasive smoothness, equalized, sense of totality, [state of infinite evenness RB]. See also *Notes*: Smoothness, all pervasive
phyam phyam	equalized, same-same
phyogs dang ris med	without time and space; nonspatial and nontemporal; impartial and nonpreferential
phyogs med	nonspatial, zero-dimensional; uni-dimensional; impartial
phyogs yan	blown wide-open; zero-dimensional; uninhibited
phyogs ris med pa	See *Notes*: Nonspatial and nontemporal
phyogs lhung med pa	indefinite, indeterminate, impartial, nontemporal and nonspatial
phrin las	perfectly appropriate activity 'phro 'dus projections; visualized
babs kyis	intrinsically, innately
babs gzhi	gratuitous ground
bya bral	nonaction. See also *Notes*: Nonaction
bya rtsol	endeavor, effort and striving [concerted effort RB]
byang chub sems	luminous mind, bodhi-mind. See also *Notes*: Luminous mind
byar med	See *Notes*: Nonaction
bying rgod	lassitude and agitation [laxity RB]
'bad rtsol	involuntarily; effortlessly
'byung 'jug	aberration, fluctuation [occurrence or involvement in RB]
dbye ba	to differentiate, define [to classify RB]

dbye bsal	differentiation or exclusion [division or exclusion RB] division or omission, sharp or blurred
dbying	spaciousness, intrinsic spaciousness [basic space RB]
ma grol ba	See *Notes*: Confinement
ma nges	indeterminate, uncertain, unpredictable. syn. nges med
ma byas	unmodified, uncontrived, unmade, unfabricated
ma yengs	non-vacillating
mi 'gyur	immutable
mi gnas	without place, unlocalized
mi rtog	unthought, nonconceptualized
mi dmigs	inconceivable, unimaginable, unobjectifiable
mi gzung	never a thing [unreified RB]
mi g.yo	unmoving, motionless
mi g.yos	unstirring, unstraying,
mi srid	not possible
dmigs bsam	critical thought, imaging [mental framework RB]
rtsal	creativity, potential [dynamic energy RB]
rtsol sgrub	striving and practicing
rtsol sgrub med	See *Notes*: Without Effort or Practice
rtsol ba med pa	undemanding, without effort
tshogs chen	great assemblage [great amassing]
mtshan ma	attributes, features, characteristics
mtshan nyid	defining characteristic
'dzin rtsol	goal-orientation, goal-fixation [reifying effort RB]
'dzin	reifying; attached, fixated
'dzin zhen	grasping, fixation
zhen pa	to crave, to fixate
zhen 'dzin	fixation
zhi ba	subside, assuage, collapse, dissolve
gzhag	disposed, settled, relaxed
bzhag	staying
zang ka ma	authentic, genuine
zang thal	boundless, transparent, unbounded
zad	resolution, exhaustion, consummation
zil gnon	outshine, overwhelm, transfigure
bzang ngan med	no better nor worse, moral judgment
bzung	reifying, attached
bzung 'dzin	See *Notes*: Dualistic perception
'ub chub	assimilated [fully embraced RB]
'ong 'gro med	pleasant and unpleasant, unvaried, invariable, unvarying
'od gsal	clear light [utterly lucid RB]
yan	unrestricted, free, expanded, unbridled, set free, let loose, run wild, total abandonment, [syn. blo bral, 'dzin med; see also rgya yan, rang yan, phyogs yan]
yang dag	immaculate, righteous
yangs dog med	without parameters
ye	See *Notes*: The now
ye klong	the matrix of the now

ye nas	in the now, timeless. See also *Notes*: The now
ye babs	disposed in the now
ye 'byams	fulfillment in the now, instant by instant suffusion [infinite expanse RB]
ye zin	holding the now
ye shes	primal~ pristine~ awareness, awareness in the now
g.yang sa	black hole, abyss, pitfall
rang ngo	original face
rang ngo shes pa	to recognize the original face
rang stong	naturally empty
rang dangs	natural radiance
rang gnas	inherent
rang babs	natural ~disposition ~state; naturally disposed, fall naturally, naturally ~occurring ~eventuating; natural state; chance; [naturally settled RB]
rang byung	self-sprung, [naturally occurring]
rang mtshan	attribute
rang yan	set free, free floating
rang rig	intrinsic presence
rang shar	arise naturally, spontaneously arising
rang zhi	collapse~ subside~ into itself
rang gzhag	left to itself, in its natural ~state ~condition, relaxed [natural rest RB]
rang bzhin	See *Notes*: Essence/nature
rang bzhin babs	naturally disposed
rang gsal	intrinsic clarity [self cognizance, self shining, natural clarity]
rig pa	pure presence, intrinsic awareness. See also *Notes*: Pure presence
ris med	nontemporal, undifferentiated, indifferent, non-preferential
la zla ba	resolve, attain finality [decisive experience RB]. See also *Notes*: Resolution
la zlos zhig	let it reach ~resolution ~completion, let it settle
las	See *Notes*: Within
lung	transmission, revelation
lhug pa	hanging loose
lhun grub	spontaneity [spontaneous presence RB]. See also *Notes*: Spontaneity
lhun mnyam	unremitting sameness, [spontaneous equalness RB]
lhun rdzogs	spontaneous perfection, spontaneously perfected
lhun yangs	ubiquitous expanse
gshis la	authenticity, natural disposition [fundamentally unconditioned state RB]
sang rgyas	See *Notes*: Buddha
bsam gtan	meditative absorption. See also *Notes*: Contemplation

Index

A

all good 2, 6-7, 33, 35-6, 52, 64-5, 69, 90
alpha-pure 7, 16, 30, 54, 64-5, 93, 104
anuyoga 16, 30, 37
atiyoga xiv-xvi, xviii, 15, 29-30, 37, 45, 57, 59

B

bodhichitta 15, 21, 50, 106.
  See also: luminous mind
buddha xix, 1, 6, 9-11, 26, 43, 67, 69, 84-6, **87-92**, 95, **104**, 106, 111 *et passim*
buddhafield(s) 6, **9-14**, 16, 26, 41, 44, **104** *et passim*

C

chos **105**, 106, 108, 109
clarity 5-6, 12, 17-18, 31, 35, 37, 40, 43, 50, 53, 56, 58, 60, 62, 70, 77, 85, 87, 108
clear light 1, 2, 9-10, 14, 17-18, 24, 30-1, 43, 50, 65, 76, 85-9, 106
compassion **21-2**, 35, 58, 80, 87, 90, 106
contemplation 82, **105**, 114
creativity xix, 5, 7, **17-19**, 21, 23, 27, 29-31, 35, **41**, 50, 52, 57, 63-6, 71, 76, 80, 85-90, 105, 111

D

dharma 26-7, 31, **105-6**, 108-9
dharmadhatu 10-11, **105-6**, 109
dharmakaya 5, 12-13, 17, **18**, 33, 36-7, **40**, 43-4, 48, 52, 62, 68, 71, 81, 90, 109
display xix, 13, 18-23, 30, 35, 40, 41, 43, 47, 66, 71, 76, 84-6, 89-90, 93, 107, 111
dualistic perception 75, **105**
Dzogchen *passim*

E

emptiness xvii, xviii, **3**, 6, 18-19, 22, 24, 39-40, 47, 58, 62, 73-4, 79, 84
experience 13-19, 21, **26-7**, 45, 52, 70, 74, 78, 81, **105** *et passim*

F

fixation 33, 47, 53-4, 61-2, 84, 85, 108
freely resting xix, **59-60**, 75, 77, 91

G

garuda xvi, xvii, 52, **88**, 89
goal-orientation xxi, 27, **29**, 55, 61, 69
guru-vision xxi, 1, 57-8, **64**, 70, 74-6, 84-5. See also: vision

Further Reading
in Radical Dzogchen

Dowman, Keith. Trans. *The Great Secret of Mind*. Ithaca, NY: Snow Lion, 2013.

_____. *Maya Yoga*, trans & comm. of Longchenpa's *Comfort and Ease in Enchantment (Sgyu ma'i ngal so)*. Kathmandu: Vajrabooks, 2010.

_____. *Old Man Basking in the Sun,* trans. & comm. of Longchenpa's *Treasury of Natural Perfection (Gnas lugs mdzod)*. Kathmandu: Vajrabooks, 2006. American Edition published as *Natural Perfection*. Boston, MA: Wisdom Publications, 2010.

_____. *Eye of the Storm,* trans. & comm. Kathmandu: Vajrabooks, 2006. Translated into German as *Im Auge des Sturms*. O.W. Barth, 2010. American edition published as *Original Perfection*. Boston, MA: Wisdom Publications, 2013.

_____. *Flight of the Garuda*, Wisdom, Boston, 1993. Translated into German as *Der Flug des Garuda* (Theseus, Zurich, 1994) and into Dutch as *De Vlucht van de Garoeda* (Uitgeveru Karnak, Amsterdam, 1994).

_____. *The Divine Madman: The Life and Songs of Drukpa Kunley*, trans., Rider & Co. London, 1982; Dawn Horse Press, U.S.A., 1983, 1998; and Pilgrim's Publishing, Kathmandu, 2000.

Dudjom Lingpa. *Buddhahood Without Meditation*. Trans. Richard Barron. Junction City, CA: Padma Publishing, 1994.

Longchen Rabjampa. *The Precious Treasury of the Basic Space of Phenomena*. Trans. Richard Barron with the Padma Translation Committee. Junction City, CA: Padma Publishing,

_____. *The Precious Treasury of the Way of Abiding*. Trans. Richard Barron with the Padma Translation Committee. Junction City, CA: Padma Publishing, 1998.

_____. *A Treasure Trove of Scriptural Transmission*. Trans. Richard Barron with the Padma Translation Committee. Junction City, CA: Padma Publishing, 2001.

Lowe, James. *Simply Being*, London, Vajra Press, 1998.

Namkhai Norbu and Adriano Clemente. *Dzogchen; The Self-Perfected State*. London: Arkana, 1989.

_____. *The Supreme Source: The Fundamental Tantra of the Dzogchen Semde*. Ithaca, NY: Snow Lion, 1995.

Nyoshul Khenpo. *Natural Great Perfection*. Trans. Surya Das. Ithaca, NY: Snow Lion, 1995.

Pema Rigtsal, Tulku. *The Great Secret of Mind*. Trans. Keith Dowman. Ithaca, N.Y: Snow Lion, 2012.

Reynolds J. *Golden Letters*. Ithaca, NY: Snow Lion, 1996.